CLIL Health Explorations

Chad Godfrey

Lauren Anderson

Frances Gleeson

Stephen O'Toole

Gautam Deshpande MD

Yoshiki Oida

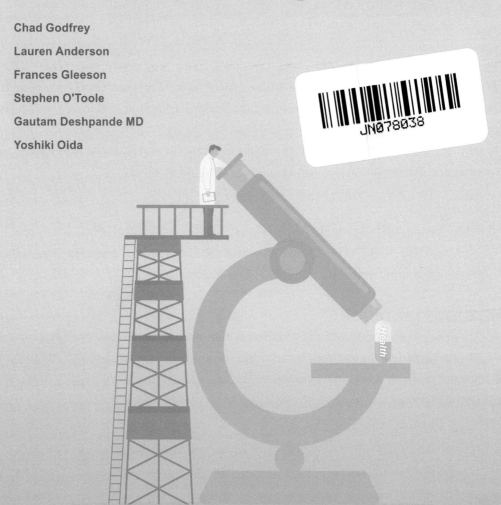

SANSHUSHA

TEXTBOOK PHILOSOPHY

CLIL Health Explorations is written for students studying healthcare at higher education institutions in Japan. The units center on pertinent health topics that are connected to their studies and will be revisited later in their professional lives.

This textbook is based on a CLIL (Content and Language Integrated Learning) framework. Each unit covers the 4Cs of CLIL (content, communication, cognition, and culture/community), while utilizing a Think-Pair-Share (TPS) learning approach. TPS gives students time to better understand content and prepare language before collaborating with their classmates. By having more time to prepare language and content, TPS can also offer students greater confidence when sharing with a partner, small groups, a larger class, or instructors. Through studying *CLIL Health Explorations*, students will have an opportunity to:

- acquire new knowledge through the textbook's content and research activities
- think and discuss about the unit's content with other students
- analyze their own country's health issues while comparing these issues with other countries
- fine-tune their language and learning skills
- produce study products based on real-world problems and/or contexts
- practice and improve poster and digital presentations

USING THIS TEXTBOOK

It is rare that a teacher finds a textbook that perfectly matches their teaching style or their students' learning styles. In addition, it's a challenge to choose a textbook that matches the students' levels in a classroom. For example, students with CEFR levels of A1/A2 may need more time to work through certain activities and will need greater language support in an EFL classroom. On the other end of the spectrum, students with high CEFR levels may need to have activities expanded to keep them motivated to use language. This textbook can be adapted to both lower and higher-level students. Although each unit is thematically based, teachers can pick and choose activities that will meet the needs of their students.

TEXTBOOK OVERVIEW

CLIL Health Explorations provides opportunities for students to work individually, in pairs, and as a small group. Through the unit activities, students research and think about information and later share their findings while checking/building their understanding with their peers. On the next page is a general overview of the textbook.

	GROUPING	ACTIVITY	SKILLS	INPUT/OUTPUT
			DAY 1	
A	Individual	What Do You Know?	Reflect on Past Knowledge	OUTPUT
B	Pair	Pair and Share #1	Communication	OUTPUT
C	Pair	Paired Listening	Listening and Communication	INPUT/OUTPUT
D	Individual	Research #1	Research	INPUT
E	Pair	Pair and Share #2	Communication	OUTPUT
F	Individual	Reading	Reading Comprehension	INPUT
G	Pair	Research #2	Research and Communication	INPUT/OUTPUT
H	Group	Research #3	Research and Communication	INPUT/OUTPUT
			DAY 2	
I	Group	Discussion	Research and Communication	INPUT/OUTPUT
J	Group	Project	Research and Project Presentation	INPUT/OUTPUT
K	Group	Presentation Skills	Varies from Unit to Unit	INPUT/OUTPUT
L	Individual	Reflection	Reflect on Lesson Learning	OUTPUT
	Ind / Pair / Gr	Unit Extensions	Varies from Unit to Unit	INPUT/OUTPUT

PRESENTATIONS

Presentations are a valuable way to synthesize knowledge and then share this knowledge with others. In addition, for EFL students, presentations are an effective way to use language while utilizing higher-order thinking skills. However, creating presentations can be a time-consuming process and lessons need to be modified based on the level of the classroom and time constraints in the class syllabus. The following is a guideline for teaching and practicing presentations in this textbook:

Units 1-7 = Poster presentations   Units 8-14 = PPT presentations

PRESENTATION ASSESSMENT, PRACTICE, AND EVALUATION

Units 1-2 / 8-9 = Assessment: Student groups create a poster/PPT with minimal teacher instruction. After presenting, instructors and classmates assess the strengths and weaknesses of the presentation and give advice.

Units 3-5 / 10-12 = Practice: Students complete a project for each of the units, but only present one of the posters/PPTs. This will give students an opportunity to practice constructing their work for each unit, and the chance to get feedback for one of their presentations as well.

Units 6-7 / 13-14 = Evaluation: Instructors choose one of the last 2 "Section J" projects and have their students complete and share a project for evaluation.

Contents

音声ダウンロード＆ストリーミングサービス（無料）のご案内

https://www.sanshusha.co.jp/text/onsei/isbn/9784384335231/

本書の音声データは、上記アドレスよりダウンロードおよびストリーミング再生ができます。ぜひご利用ください。

Download

Streaming

Health and Nutrition

Ⓐ What Do You Know?

What do you know about nutrition? Write 3 ideas below.

1) _____

_____

2) _____

_____

3) _____

_____

Ⓑ Pair and Share #1

Talk with a partner and share your ideas from Section A. Remember to ask follow-up questions or make comments as your partner shares their answers:

- I've heard about…
- Why do you think that?
- Me, too! / That's what I think! / I wrote the same idea!
- Oh really? I have some different answers.

Ⓒ Paired Listening

001
1-1

a) Work with a partner. Listen to a classroom teacher talk about how diets have changed over time. Take notes as you listen and answer the questions below.

1) What were diets like in the past?
2) In what way have diets recently changed?

b) Work with a partner and check your answers.

EXTENSIONS ➡ What are some good points about our modern diet?

_____

_____

Some foods are considered unhealthy because they lack nutrition. What are 10 foods that are considered to be bad for your health if eaten as a regular part of your diet? Research online and make a list below. Do NOT forget to include why the food is unhealthy.

Unhealthy Food	Why Is It Unhealthy?
1)	
2)	
3)	
4)	
5)	
6)	
7)	
8)	
9)	
10)	

E Pair and Share #2

Compare your answers from Section D with a classmate. Which answers are the same? Which answers are different? Discuss and decide which food is the UNHEALTHIEST on each of your lists. Give reasons to support your thinking.

A: I think cakes and cookies are the worst because they contain a lot of sugar, refined flour, and trans fats. Which one did you choose?

B: I have a different opinion. I chose soft drinks. From the research I did online, I found that soft drinks are mostly sugar and can raise a person's risk for diabetes and heart disease.

EXTENSIONS ➡ What do you think is the unhealthiest Japanese food? Why?

_____

_____

F **Reading – Health and Nutrition**

Nutrition is important for all plants and animals. For humans, the building blocks of life come from nutrients in food. Food nutrients are the fuel that keeps our bodies running smoothly. **Carbohydrates**, proteins, and fats, as well as vitamins and minerals, are all needed to keep our bodies healthy. However, not just any kind of food will keep our bodies in good

5　shape. A diet rich in whole grains, like brown rice and whole wheat, and a variety of fruits and vegetables is important. Lean meats and fish are full of protein, but so are foods like legumes, lentils, and soy products, like tofu. Therefore, eating healthy and having a diet full of the right nutrients seems easy, right? Well, in our modern world, it may not be so easy.

We need a good balance of nutrients in the food we eat. Carbohydrates are important for

10　energy but we need healthy carbohydrates like whole grains, nuts, and fresh fruits and vegetables. Carbohydrates that are low in nutrients, like white sugar, refined white bread, or processed foods, provide "**empty calories**" and can **lead to** unhealthy outcomes. The same is true for fats. Healthy fats like omega-3 or omega-6 fatty acids come from olive oil, different kinds of fish, nuts, and soybeans. Trans fats are a type of fat to avoid. These unhealthy fats can

15　be found in a lot of highly processed foods like mass-produced baked goods, margarine, and non-dairy coffee creamer.

How much of each nutrient should we have in our daily diet? There is no easy answer to this question; it depends on the individual (for example, young or old, male or female). As a general guideline, about 10% - 25% of your daily calories should come from protein, around

20　10% from fats, and the rest of your calories should come from healthy carbohydrates. However, some people do not follow these guidelines and end up eating too many empty calories each day. This can have an effect on your entire body, contributing to problems like **obesity** and lifestyle diseases like diabetes, high cholesterol, and cardiovascular disease.

Your digestive tract (also called your gastrointestinal tract or GI tract) works to move

25　and process all the food and liquid you consume. As it breaks down food into smaller parts, your body absorbs nutrients. Your large intestine absorbs water, and the waste products of digestion become the stool that is pushed out through the anus. It is important to note that the digestive system is complex. Digestive disorders or diseases can occur when an organ is not functioning well. Some problems that occur with the digestive system can be connected

30　to obesity. **Gastroesophageal reflux disease (GERD), chronic constipation, irritable bowel syndrome (IBS)**, and stomach cancer are some examples.

Obesity is rapidly becoming a worldwide **epidemic**. It is one of the leading causes of death worldwide. Even though Japan still has a low obesity rate, it is steadily increasing especially among middle-aged men. It was reported that the number of overweight Japanese

35　men with a body mass index (BMI) of 25 or greater was 33% in 2019.

carbohydrates (carbs) 炭水化物
empty calories カロリー不足
lead to ～に導く
obese/obesity 肥満の／肥満

gastroesophageal reflux disease (GERD) 逆流性食道炎
chronic constipation 慢性の便秘
irritable bowel syndrome (IBS) 過敏症腸症候群
epidemic 伝染性の

Language Point | **Nonreversible Word Pairs**

Some word pairs in English appear in a fixed order. If they are reversed, they can sound odd. Some examples include:

- fruits and vegetables
- salt and pepper
- cream and sugar / milk and sugar
- fish and chips
- bread and butter

G Research #2 – Anatomy

a) Work alone. Label the parts of the digestive system below. If you do NOT know an answer, leave it blank. NOTE In part (a) do NOT look online for the answers.

b) After, work with a partner and discuss your answers. Fill in any of the answers you are missing.

c) Next, work with your partner and check your answers online.

d) Finally, your teacher will give you the answers. Check to see if your answers are correct.

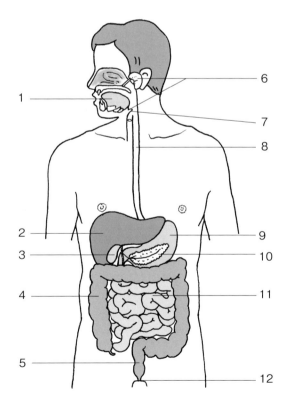

1) _____
2) _____
3) _____
4) _____
5) _____
6) _____
7) _____
8) _____
9) _____
10) _____
11) _____
12) _____

H Research #3 – Group Work

Make a team of 3-4 members. Choose one organ from Section G and research its function. After each team is finished, share your answers.

Organ's name: _____

Important functions:

_____

_____

EXTENSIONS Gastroesophageal reflux disease (GERD) is a common health problem. What is GERD? What are the symptoms? What is the treatment? Research online and find the answers.

_____

_____

I Discussion – Should Junk Food Be Banned?

"Junk food" refers to foods low in nutrition, high in sugar and/or fat, and high in calories. Most people eat junk food from time to time. It tastes good and is often cheap. However, junk food is also causing many health problems worldwide. What is your opinion about junk food? Is it good or is it bad? Is it so bad that it should be banned (made illegal)?

Work with a team of 3-4 members. Discuss the good points about junk food and the bad points. After discussing, vote in your team to ban or not ban junk food. Then, compare your vote with the rest of the class. NOTE Be ready to give reasons for your choice.

Good Points	Bad Points

J Project – Diets

a) **Work with a team of 3-4 members. Choose one kind of diet from the list below and research about it.**

☐ Mediterranean diet   ☐ Japanese diet   ☐ Vegetarianism

☐ Veganism   ☐ Paleo diet   ☐ Low-carb diet

☐ Intermittent fasting   ☐ Raw food diet   ☐ Ketogenic diet

b) **Create a team poster to share what you learned. Include the following information on your poster:**

- What is the definition of the diet you chose? • What foods does it include?
- What are the pros and cons of this diet?
- How does it benefit or harm the digestive system?
- Include photos, illustrations, and/or diagrams to support your research.
- Include references, showing where you found the information online.

K Presentation Skills – Stage Fright

Many people have a fear of public speaking. Face it, everyone feels some anxiety when speaking to a group of people whether the group is large or small. What can you do to reduce your stage fright in your next presentation? Below are 5 tips:

1) Make friends with the audience before your talk. Arrive early for your presentation, smile, greet, and speak with audience members as they arrive.

2) Be organized! Plan what you will do, in the order you need to do it in.

3) Practice several times before your scheduled presentation (see Unit 7).

4) Breathe deeply and get centered. Don't let your nervousness dominate you. Get your emotions under control by deep breathing and giving yourself positive and confident advice before your talk.

5) Remember that the audience is on your side; they are cheering for you to do well.

EXTENSIONS ➡

a) **Work with the same team members from Section J.**
b) **Put your team's poster on the wall.**
c) **Do "Rock, Paper, Scissors."**
d) **The winner: Stand 1 meter away and share information for 1 minute. After, rank your level of stage fright from 1-10 ("1" being relaxed to "10" being very anxious).**
e) **Discuss with your team members what you can do to reduce your level of stage fright.**
f) **Repeat until each team member has had a chance to practice.**

L Reflection

Work alone. Think back over what you have learned in this unit and record your answers below.

1) What are some interesting things you have learned in this unit?
2) What do you want to improve about your learning?
3) If you did a presentation, what went well? What did not?

Unit 2

Fitness and Exercise

Ⓐ What Do You Know?

What do you know about fitness and exercise? Write 3 ideas below.

1) _____

_____

2) _____

_____

3) _____

_____

Ⓑ Pair and Share #1

Talk with a partner and share your ideas from Section A. Remember to ask follow-up questions or make comments as your partner shares their answers:

- Interesting!
- That's unbelievable!
- I never knew that!
- I've never heard of that.

Ⓒ Paired Listening

a) Work with a partner. Listen to a doctor talking to her patient. Take notes as you listen and answer the questions below.

1) What is the patient's BMI?
2) What parts of the body does the patient mention getting injured?
3) Why doesn't the patient want to go to the gym?
4) What types of activities does the doctor suggest for the patient to avoid injury?

b) Work with a partner and check your answers.

EXTENSIONS ➡ Do you regularly exercise? What kind of exercise do you do? What is the hardest physical exercise you have ever done?

_____

_____

What are the benefits of regular exercise and what are the possible consequences of NOT exercising regularly? Research online and make a list below.

Benefits of Regular Exercise	Consequences of Insufficient Exercise
1)	1)
2)	2)
3)	3)
4)	4)
5)	5)
6)	6)
7)	7)
8)	8)
9)	9)
10)	10)

E **Pair and Share #2**

Compare your answers from Section D with a classmate. Which answers are the same? Which answers are different? Which of the benefits in Section D are the most important? In terms of exercise, do you think you lead a more healthy or less healthy life than your partner? Give reasons to support your thinking.

A: I believe that the greatest benefit is you can boost your endurance. Also, I think I am healthier because I belong to the swimming club. I train two times a week.

B: I think you are healthy but not healthier than me. I also belong to a sports club. I play soccer four times a week. I benefit from muscle training.

EXTENSIONS ➡ What could you do to improve your fitness? What new physical activity could you do to make your life healthier?

_____

_____

F Reading – Fitness and Exercise

We all know that exercise is good for you, and following a physically active lifestyle can prove beneficial to many facets of your life. Exercise can improve your health both physically and mentally. Not only does regular exercise control weight, it also improves blood **circulation**. Exercise contributes to sending a variety of beneficial chemical and physical signals to tissues
5   that help reduce inflammation and optimize metabolic functioning.

Good blood circulation is also important to the white blood cells in your immune system. In other words, physical activity helps your body defend itself better and avoid potential diseases and sickness. The right amount of regular exercise also increases high-density **lipoprotein (HDL)**. This is often called "good" **cholesterol** and can help regulate
10   more dangerous types of fats in the body. For example, optimal levels of HDL can help keep **triglycerides** and low-density lipoprotein (**LDL**) cholesterol within safe levels, reducing the risk of **cardiovascular** diseases. It can also help prevent other vital organs such as the **pancreas**, **liver**, and **kidneys** from becoming **vulnerable** to disease.

In addition, engaging in moderate amounts of regular exercise and using stored energy
15   may actually boost one's energy level rather than deplete it. Having improved energy allows us to go about daily activities with a better positivity, which leads to additional benefits for mental health. Common psychological benefits gained through exercise include increased satisfaction in oneself, a pride in physical achievements, improved self-esteem, and improved mood and outlook—all of which can reduce stress and decrease symptoms associated with
20   mental illness, such as depression.

Conversely, neglecting to exercise and failure to engage in regular physical activities increases the risk of obesity, which may lead to **metabolic syndrome**. There is also a greater possibility of type 2 diabetes mellitus and a higher chance of several cardiovascular diseases. A lack of exercise can also induce **fatigue** and an overall **lethargy**, difficulty in sleeping, and
25   increase the risk of depression. Ultimately, an inactive lifestyle increases the risk of more severe **morbidity** and earlier **mortality**—the consequences do not get any more serious than that!

> **Words and Phrases**
>
> circulation （血液の）循環
> lipoprotein リポタンパク質
> HDL 高密度リポタンパク質
> cholesterol コレステロール
> triglycerides トリグリセリド
> LDL 低密度リポタンパク質
> cardiovascular 循環器の
> pancreas 膵臓
>
> liver 肝臓
> kidneys 腎臓
> vulnerable （人・体などが）傷つきやすい
> metabolic syndrome メタボリック症候群
> fatigue 疲労、倦怠感
> lethargy 倦怠、脱力感
> morbidity 病的な状態
> mortality 死亡率

Collocations are a group of two or more words that are used naturally together. Examples from the reading passage include:

- increase the risk/reduce the risk
- a greater possibility
- a higher chance
- a lack of exercise

G Research #2 – Anatomy

a) Work alone. First, label various parts of the body. After, list one or more injuries that may occur to that body part through exercise or sport. NOTE In part (a) do NOT look online for the answers.
b) After, work with a partner and discuss your answers. Fill in any of the answers you are missing.
c) Next, work with your partner and check your answers online.
d) Finally, your teacher will give you the answers. Check to see if your answers are correct.

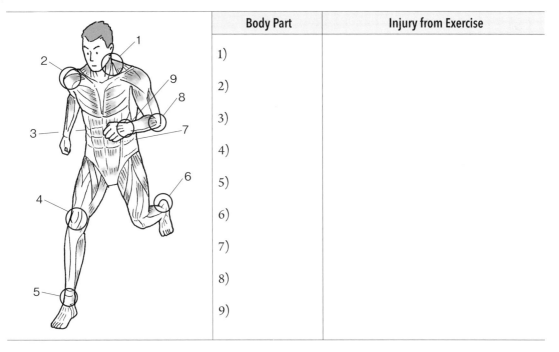

	Body Part	Injury from Exercise
1)		
2)		
3)		
4)		
5)		
6)		
7)		
8)		
9)		

H Research #3 – Group Work

Make a team of 3-4 members. Research the function of one of the body parts from Section G, and why it is important in exercise. After each team is finished, share your answers.

Body part: _____

Important functions:

_____

_____

Why is it important in exercise?:

_____

_____

_____

EXTENSIONS ➡ Did you know there is such a thing as overexercising or overtraining? Studies have shown that overexercising may not only be counterproductive but also can actually be dangerous. Research online and find out more about the side effects of overexercising.

_____

_____

Ⓘ Discussion – Should Exercise Be Compulsory at Universities and the Workplace?

Whether part of school curricula, in extracurricular competition, or simply in play, most school-age children engage in an adequate amount of physical activity. However, as we get older we tend to have less time, less opportunities, and less motivation to exercise. In addition to this, too often people realize this to be the case only after a medical problem due to inactivity has occurred. Should university students or employees of a company be forced to exercise? What are some potential advantages of this? Are there any disadvantages and, if so, what would they be?

Work with a team of 3-4 members. Discuss the good and bad points of compulsory exercise for adults. After discussing, vote in your team whether you think it is a good idea or a bad idea to make exercise compulsory. Then, compare your vote with the rest of the class. NOTE Be ready to give reasons for your choice.

Good Points of Compulsory Exercise	Bad Points of Compulsory Exercise

Ⓙ Project – Exercise, Fitness, and Sport

a) Work with a team of 3-4 members. Choose one kind of exercise or sport and research about it.
b) Create a poster promoting good health through the exercise or sport your team has chosen.
c) Talk about the positive effects it can have on the human body and mind, and why people should choose this form of exercise over others.
d) Include the following information on your poster:

- What is the name of the exercise or sport, and what kind of activity is it?
- What are the benefits to the individual?　　• Are there any social benefits?
- Are there any risks associated with this activity?
- Include photos, illustrations, and/or diagrams to support your research.
- Include references showing where you found the information online.

Presentation Skills – Planning a Presentation

Getting started is probably the most difficult thing when considering making a presentation. Once you have your idea or theme for the presentation, what comes next? Below are some tips for planning your presentation:

1) Brainstorming – There are several ways to brainstorm including mind mapping, listing, or making Venn diagrams. Choose the method that best suits your theme.

2) Timing – How long is your presentation? 5 minutes? 10 minutes? 20 minutes? This will impact on how long your script will be.

3) Research – Once you have the framework, you can start to research the relevant topics. When researching, start first on gathering information that will support the most important points you want to make.

4) Structure – Ideas and information need to be presented in a logical order so that your presentation flows well.

5) Script writing – Language suitability is very important. Who is your audience (e.g., professors, students, patients)?

6) Transitions – Think about the best way to link your ideas and move from one point to the next.

7) Visual component – Whether making slides or a poster, decide how many slides you will need or the layout of the poster.

8) Editing – It is ok to add or remove information as the process evolves.

EXTENSIONS **➡ Work with the same team members from Section J. Look back at Section J. Did you follow each of the points?**

Theme: Did you identify what you are going to talk about?

Brainstorm: Did you choose the method that best suits your theme?

Timing: Did you aim for the correct amount of time?

Research: Did you research the most relevant topics?

Structure: Did you put your ideas into a logical order?

Script: Did you consider your audience?

Transitions: Did you use transitional phrases between your points while you were speaking?

Visual component: Did you consider the layout of your slides or poster before you started to construct your visual?

Editing: What will you change in terms of the order or additional information?

 Reflection

Work alone. Think back over what you have learned in this unit and record your answers below.

1) What are some interesting things you have learned in this unit?

2) What do you want to improve about your learning?

3) If you did a presentation, what went well? What did not?

The Skeletal System and Orthopedic Disorders

A What Do You Know?

What do you know about the skeletal system or orthopedic disorders? Write 3 ideas below.

1) _____

_____

2) _____

_____

3) _____

_____

B Pair and Share #1

Talk with a partner and share your ideas from Section A. Remember to ask follow-up questions or make comments as your partner shares their answers:

- That's (really) amazing!
- Why do you think that?
- I have that same answer! / That's interesting, but I wrote about...
- Another thing I've heard is...

C Paired Listening

005 1-5

a) Work with a partner. Listen to a doctor talk about lowering your risk of losing bone density. Take notes as you listen and answer the questions below.

1) What can happen to our bones as we age?
2) What should you do if one of your family members has osteoporosis?
3) What do you need to make vitamin D work in your body?
4) What are 3 other preventable risk factors that can lower bone density?

b) Work with a partner and check your answers.

EXTENSIONS ➡ Do you have a sedentary lifestyle? Do you spend a lot of your time sitting or do you balance your sitting time with exercise or activity?

_____

_____

D Research #1 – Which Foods Are Good for Your Bones? Which Foods Are Not?

Promoting good bone health by eating the right balance of foods is important. Avoiding heavy consumption of foods that may cause lower bone density is equally important. Research online and find out more about the foods that are good for your bones and the ones that are not. Make a list below.

Foods That Are Good for Bone Health	Foods That Are NOT Good for Bone Health
1)	1)
2)	2)
3)	3)
4)	4)
5)	5)

E Pair and Share #2

Compare your answers from Section D with a classmate. Which answers are the same? Which answers are different? Looking at your diet, which of the above foods in Section D do you think you could eat more to have healthier bones? Which ones could you eat less? Give reasons to support your thinking.

A: I don't like milk, so I feel I need something else to keep my bones healthy. I decided to eat more soy products and reduce the number of soft drinks I drink.

B: I think my diet is pretty good, but I think I should be outdoors more to help process the vitamin D from my diet.

EXTENSIONS ➡ In general, when comparing the bones of modern humans with early hunter-gatherers, our bones have become weaker. Why do you think that this has happened?

_____

_____

F Reading – The Skeletal System and Orthopedic Disorders

Take a moment and imagine your body without a skeletal system. You would look something like a **jellyfish**! Our bones are very important in many ways. They give us support, help us stand upright, carry our weight, protect vital organs from harm, and work together with muscles to give us structure and allow for movement. Our bones also perform another
5   important job: they help produce red and white blood cells. Below are some other interesting facts about our bones:

- The skeletal system is made up of around 300 bones at birth, but later many of these bones **fuse** together, leaving us with 206 as adults.
- There are a lot of bones in your hand (27 in each of them) and in your foot as well (26
10   in each).
- The largest bone in the body is your **femur**, while the smallest are the three bones located in your ears (the **malleus**, **incus**, and **stapes**).
- Your bones stop growing in length around **puberty**, but their strength and density will continue to change throughout your life.

15   The quality of your diet and daily exercise are important to strengthen and maintain bone health. Foods that are rich in calcium, vitamin D, and other nutrients can help to improve your bone density. A balanced diet including natural sources of fruits and vegetables (especially some kinds of green leafy vegetables), nuts, tofu, lean meats, fish, and dairy products are just a few choices to keep your bones in great shape. However, foods that are
20   high in **oxalates** (like fresh spinach) and **phytates** (like wheat bran) may interfere with calcium absorption from other foods. These are healthy foods, but be careful how you pair them with foods that promote bone health.

Along with diet, exercise is key to keeping your bones strong and preventing bone density loss. Regular weight-bearing exercises like jogging, tennis, dancing, jumping rope,
25   hiking, and stair climbing, are just some of the ways to be physically active and keep your bones from losing mass. Exercising for about 30 minutes a day, about 3-4 times a week is recommended. For the elderly, regular exercise is most important. Bones lose mass as we get older, so having a **sedentary**, indoor lifestyle can speed up adverse effects on bone health.

Osteoporosis is a disease which literally means "**porous** bone." It is a condition where
30   your bones lose strength and lose mass. It is often called "the silent disease" because you may not know you have it until a bone breaks. It can affect all genders and races, but affects Asian and white women the most and especially post-**menopausal** women, who are at a higher risk. Worldwide, it is reported that 1 in 3 women and 1 in 5 men over the age of 50 will suffer from a broken bone because of osteoporosis. Signs and symptoms might include back pain,
35   loss of height, a **stooped** posture, and bones that break easily.

jellyfish クラゲ	stapes （中耳の）あぶみ骨	osteoporosis 骨粗しょう症
fuse 融合する、一緒になる	puberty 思春期	porous 多孔質の、透過性の
femur 大腿骨	oxalates シュウ酸塩［エステル］	menopausal 閉経後の
malleus （中耳の）つち骨	phytates フィチン酸塩	stooped 前かがみの、猫背の
incus きぬた骨	sedentary 座っている	

Language Point   **Medical Mnemonics**

A mnemonic is a memory device to remember information. In medicine there are many mnemonics to help remember complex medical knowledge. Here is an example to remember the 8 small bones that make up the wrist (carpal bones):

Sally **L**eft **T**he **P**arty **T**o **T**ake **C**athy **H**ome

Scaphoid, **L**unate, **T**riquetrum, **P**isiform, **T**rapezium, **T**rapezoid, **C**apitate, and **H**amate

G   **Research #2 – Anatomy**

a) Work alone. Label the 6 bone classifications below. If you do NOT know an answer, leave it blank.
    NOTE In part (a) do NOT look online for the answers.

b) After, work with a partner and discuss your answers. Fill in any of the answers you are missing.

c) Next, work with your partner and check your answers online.

d) Finally, your teacher will give you the answers. Check to see if your answers are correct.

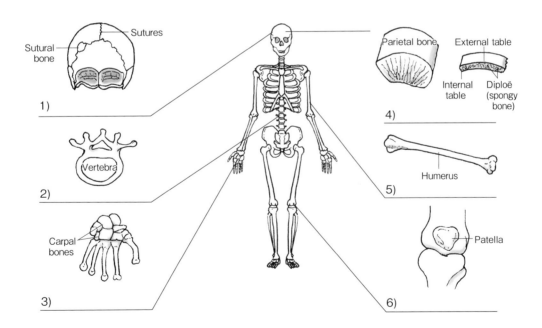

Sutures
Sutural bone
1)
Vertebra
2)
Carpal bones
3)
Parietal bone   External table
Internal table   Diploë (spongy bone)
4)
Humerus
5)
Patella
6)

H   Research #3 – Group Work

Make a team of 3-4 members. Choose one bone disorder from the box below and research the 3 following points. After each team is finished, share your answers.

Types of Bone Disorders (choose one):

☐ Paget's disease   ☐ rheumatoid arthritis   ☐ scoliosis   ☐ locomotive syndrome
☐ gout   ☐ bursitis   ☐ rickets   ☐ osteonecrosis

Definition:

_____

_____

Signs / Symptoms:

_____

_____

Treatment:

_____

_____

EXTENSIONS ➡ Diabetes can increase the risk of various bone and joint problems. Research online and find out more.

_____

_____

I   Discussion – Is Drinking Milk Necessary to Build Stronger Bones?

Some say that we must drink milk for strong bone health while others disagree. What do you think?

a) Your teacher will assign your team either a pro or con position. Research and discuss your position on whether drinking milk is needed for strong bones (pro) or not (con). Be ready to give reasons for your choices.

Pros	Cons
1)	1)
2)	2)
3)	3)
4)	4)
5)	5)

b) After a team presents one of their position points, the other team needs to offer a rebuttal point. Teams continue until they have shared all their position points. NOTE Throughout the discussion, be sure to take notes on the other teams' positions.

c) After the discussion, do a class vote: Which side of the debate do you agree with and why?

Project – Osteoporosis Prevention Poster

a) Work with a team of 3-4 members.
b) Create an information poster on the topic of osteoporosis prevention.
c) First, share and take notes about the ideas that you have learned from this unit. After, research online and find more information.
d) Select and organize the most important information you have collected for your poster.
e) Plan the pictures, illustrations, diagrams, and text for your poster, and then complete a final draft of your poster.
f) Include references showing where you found the information online.

 Presentation Skills – Research Poster Layouts

Presenting a research poster is a good way to share information with a small audience. Although a conference may provide guidelines for your poster layout, these are some general guidelines that can help make your poster visually effective:
1) Create a title that catches a person's attention.
2) Make sure the author(s) names are prominent after the title.
3) Divide the information on your poster in vertical columns.
4) Keep your word count around 1000 words to avoid clutter on your poster.
5) Use fonts that can be seen 1 meter away.
6) Use boldface headings and spaces between your sections so that the reader can follow the flow of your poster.
7) Use bullets and numbering to make your poster easy to read.
8) Avoid using busy or bright color backgrounds. Instead, use colors that contrast.
9) Make sure your tables and figures cover only about 50% of the poster's area.
10) Include your email address (or QR code) and references at the end. Including your contact information is useful if you are away from your poster during a conference.

EXTENSIONS ➡

a) Work with the same team members from Section J.
b) From the list above, which of these 10 points does your poster cover? Which points have been left out?
c) Discuss in your team how to make your poster ready for an academic conference; what does your team need to do to improve your poster?

 Reflection

Work alone. Think back over what you have learned in this unit and record your answers below.

1) What are some interesting things you have learned in this unit?
2) What do you want to improve about your learning?
3) If you did a presentation, what went well? What did not?

Chronic Diseases

Ⓐ What Do You Know?

What do you know about chronic diseases? Write 3 ideas below.

1) _____

_____

2) _____

_____

3) _____

_____

Ⓑ Pair and Share #1

Talk with a partner and share your ideas from Section A. Remember to ask follow-up questions or make comments as your partner shares their answers:

- That's fascinating!
- Tell me more. Why do you think so?
- Some people say…
- Nice! Not only that, but I also wrote about…

Ⓒ Paired Listening

[007 1-7]

a) Work with a partner. Listen to a classroom teacher talk about chronic diseases. Take notes as you listen and answer the questions below.

1) What are some of the most common chronic diseases?
2) Are chronic diseases always the result of an unhealthy lifestyle?

b) Work with a partner and check your answers.

[EXTENSIONS] ➡ Do you think the incidence of chronic disease will continue to increase in the future? Why?

_____

_____

Living with long-term illnesses can be both physically and mentally exhausting for patients. Research online and make a list of 10 chronic diseases below. After, look online and list the possible treatments for each illness. (As some diseases will have common treatments, try to come up with as many different answers for treatment possibilities as you can.)

Chronic Diseases	Treatments
1)	
2)	
3)	
4)	
5)	
6)	
7)	
8)	
9)	
10)	

E **Pair and Share #2**

Compare your answers from Section D with a classmate. Which answers are the same? Which answers are different? Discuss and decide which chronic disease is the easiest to cope with. Give reasons to support your thinking.

A: I think asthma is one of the easiest chronic diseases to manage. Inhalers allow most people with asthma to lead an active life.

B: I have a different opinion. I chose psoriasis, because in most cases it doesn't have a high risk of death.

EXTENSIONS ➡ What do you think is the most common chronic illness in Japan? Why?

_____

_____

008
1-8

Over the past few decades, the **prevalence** of chronic diseases that adversely affect **quality of life (QOL)** has steadily increased. Dealing with poor health over time can take an emotional toll, robbing patients of their personal **autonomy** and hope for the future. The Centers for Disease Control and Prevention (CDC) defines quality of life as an individual's
5 perceived physical and mental health over time. Measuring QOL generally falls into three key areas: physical, psychological, and social functioning. People living with chronic diseases need more support in these three areas to help them better manage their long-term illnesses.

Chronic disease is a leading factor in limiting **mobility**. In a study of twins between the ages of 71 and 75, the disease-free individuals took around 7000 steps a day, whereas those
10 with chronic illnesses accrued less than 4000 steps. Making appropriate exercise choices is an important factor in avoiding further injury or disability; for example, a healthcare provider might suggest that a patient with joint disease integrate **low-impact aerobic exercises** that are easier on joints such as walking or swimming. Tailoring exercise therapies to the type of disease can significantly improve individuals physical functioning, mobility, and possibilities
15 for independent living.

Studies on QOL have shown that chronic illness has a negative effect on mental health and increases the incidence of depression. There is a risk of a downward spiral in which a patient may discontinue treatments, becoming more depressed as their health rapidly declines. Studies have found that the incidence of mental health problems among patients living with a
20 chronic disease varies with age, gender, and **socioeconomic status**; participants older than 70 years, women, and people in the lowest wealth brackets are more likely to suffer from depression. According to a study, people who have a high sense of control tended to mentally cope well with chronic illness, displaying reduced distress and higher self-worth. To promote a positive mindset in patients, the study advocates for **psychotherapy** alongside regular
25 medical appointments, as well as daily journaling to better observe stressors or facilitate improvements in symptoms.

Chronic illness can influence a person's ability to work, negatively affecting patients financially while alienating them from society. Mobility issues and a higher incidence of depression may result in patients withdrawing from friends, family, and social activities.
30 **Meta-studies** on managing long-term disease have shown that having good relationships is the number one factor in coping with chronic illness. A strong social network can mean that symptoms are noticed earlier; patients are also more likely to be encouraged to eat healthy food or exercise more. Conversely, having people who depend on them can encourage patients to take care of themselves and better manage their illness. Another study found that **social**
35 **engagement** can enhance disease management and prevent a chronic condition from progressing to disability.

To help ensure the best QOL for their patients, it is crucial that healthcare providers not only aim to improve physical health, but promote interventions to **stave off** mental illness and increase social engagement amongst the chronically ill.

Words and Phrases

prevalence 蔓延、有病率	socioeconomic status 社会経済的な地位
quality of life (QOL) 生活の質	psychotherapy 精神療法
autonomy 自律性	meta-studies メタ研究
mobility 移動性、可動性	social engagement 社会的関与
low-impact aerobic exercise 身体に負担の少ない有酸素運動	stave off 〜を避ける、免れる

Language Point   British and American English

There are some differences between British and American English medical terms. Here are some common differences:

British English	American English
A&E (Accident and Emergency)	ER (Emergency Room)
operating theatre	operating room
chemist/pharmacy	drug store/pharmacy
jab (flu jab, booster jab)	shot (flu shot, booster shot)
tablets	pills
plaster	Band-aid

G Research #2 – Anatomy

a) Work alone. Look at the list of chronic diseases. Write down the part(s) of the body that are affected by the chronic diseases. If you do NOT know an answer, leave it blank. NOTE In part (a) do NOT look online for the answers.

b) After, work with a partner and discuss your answers. Fill in any of the answers you are missing.

c) Next, work with your partner and check your answers online.

d) Finally, your teacher will give you the answers. Check to see if your answers are correct.

Part(s) of the Body	Chronic Diseases
	Alzheimer's disease, Parkinson's disease, ALS (Lou Gehrig's disease), epilepsy
	asthma, chronic obstructive pulmonary disease (COPD), cystic fibrosis
	stroke, hypertension, angina
	cataracts, glaucoma, age-related macular degeneration (AMD)
	osteoporosis, scoliosis, osteoarthritis
	psoriasis, acne, rosacea

H Research #3 – Group Work

Make a team of 3-4 members. Choose one chronic disease from Section G and research its signs and symptoms. After each team is finished, share your answers.

Name: _____

Signs/Symptoms: _____

_____

_____

EXTENSIONS ➔ Of the chronic diseases discussed by all the groups, which one do you think is the most serious? Why? Research online and find the answers.

_____

_____

I Discussion – Do Plant-based Diets Reduce the Risk of Chronic Disease?

There are several types of plant-based diets, such as vegetarian and vegan diets. Most vegetarian diets exclude fish and meat (and sometimes eggs), while vegan diets also exclude foods produced from animals, such as cheese, honey, and gelatin. There is a growing debate that a link may exist between chronic disease and diets high in animal products. What is your opinion? Should people adopt a plant-based diet to avoid long-term illnesses?

Work with a team of 3-4 members. Research and discuss the health benefits of plant-based diets and omnivorous (including both animal and plant-based food) diets. After discussing, decide with your team if a plant-based diet is the best option for reducing the risk of chronic disease.

Support for Plant-based Diets	Support for an Omnivorous Diets

Project – Is There Anything You Can Do This Week to Improve Your Health?

Imagine you are a patient suffering from a chronic disease. Your doctor asks you, "Is there anything you can do this week to improve your health?" How would you answer?

Create a poster to share your response. Include the following information in your poster:

- My chronic disease is _____
- What will I do this week to improve my health?
- How will the activity/lifestyle change be modified for my chronic disease?
- What are the general benefits of this activity/lifestyle change?
- How could this activity/lifestyle change benefit my chronic disease?
- How will I measure my progress?

 Presentation Skills – Research Skills

Imagine you have finished the planning and brainstorming for your presentation. Next, you need to find the information that supports your theme. This is the research stage. Below you will find some tips to help you research more effectively:

1) Choose one point about your research topic and start creating questions.
2) Search the internet – type in one term or key in one of your questions. Scroll down the list of search results.
3) Make sure you get information from reliable websites. One method is to check the domain suffixes. (e.g., .com/.gov/.edu/.org)
4) Get information from more than one website and compare the information. As you find good information, copy and paste the link into a prepared document titled "References."
5) When taking notes be careful not to copy information. Look for the main ideas and write them in your own words and change the verbs and nouns to similar meaning words. Do not cut and paste!
6) Organize your notes effectively using dates, headings, and sub-headings.

EXTENSIONS
a) Look back at your work for Unit 3, page 25, Section J.
b) Review your research work for Section J. Did you follow the advice above?
c) Which points did you follow well? Which ones do you need to improve?

 Reflection

Work alone. Think back over what you have learned in this unit and record your answers below.

1) What are some interesting things you have learned in this unit?
2) What do you want to improve about your learning?
3) If you did a presentation, what went well? What did not?

Unit 5 Cancer

A What Do You Know?

What do you know about how cancer affects people? Write 3 ideas below.

1) _____

_____

2) _____

_____

3) _____

_____

B Pair and Share #1

Talk with a partner and share your ideas from Section A. Remember to ask follow-up questions or make comments as your partner shares their answers:

- I didn't know that!
- You probably heard that...
- Would you mind repeating that?
- That sounds (pretty) serious.

C Paired Listening

a) Work with a partner. Listen to a university professor talk about the history of cancer. Take notes as you listen and answer the questions below.

1) Does cancer have a long history?
2) Is cancer a human-made disease?
3) Where have the earliest examples of cancer in humans been found?
4) Why is the incidence of cancer increasing in our modern world?

b) Work with a partner and check your answers.

EXTENSIONS ➥ What is the origin of the word "cancer"? Research online and find the answer.

_____

_____

D Research #1 – Causes of Cancer

The causes of cancer are complex. Research online and find out more about some of the known causes of cancer. Make a list of these causes below.

Known Causes of Cancer
1)
2)
3)
4)
5)
6)
7)
8)
9)
10)

E Pair and Share #2

Compare your answers from Section D with a classmate. Which answers are the same? Which answers are different? Looking at your lifestyle, discuss and decide which of the above causes are preventable. Give reasons to support your thinking.

A: I think I could start exercising more. Lately, I just spend time on my smartphone or watching TV in the evening.

B: Yeah, me too. I also think I should change my diet. I eat too many processed meats like sausage and ham.

EXTENSIONS ➡ In Japan, which of the above do you think are the top 3 preventable causes of cancer? Give reasons to support your choices.

010
1-10

Cancer has a long history. The earliest description of cancer dates back to the times of the Egyptians in 3000 BCE. The origin of the word is connected to the Greek physician, Hippocrates. He used the terms *carcinos* and *carcinoma* to describe cancer. These two words are related to the word "crab" in Greek because of the shape of the disease as it spreads in the body.

5

Cancer is a **non-communicable** disease (NCD), and the second leading cause of death worldwide. Cancer starts with a **mutation** in a cell's DNA which, in turn, leads to mutated **genes**. Normal genes tell the cell what to do—how to act, how to divide, how to grow, and when to die. Mutations are always occurring as genes replicate; most mutations have no effects on health, and some can even be beneficial. However, once a cancer-causing mutation happens in a gene, several things can occur: it can tell the cell to grow more rapidly with the same mutated gene; fail to stop mutated cells from growing in large numbers; and make mistakes in repairing DNA errors. These gene mutations can either be something you are born with or may be acquired after birth from any number of outside influences (for example, from smoking, diet, or environmental **pollutants**).

10

15

Who is at risk for getting cancer? First, it is important to note that most risk factors do not directly cause cancer. One person, even with several risk factors, may never develop cancer, while another person with no risk factors might develop the disease. In addition, when it comes to the risk of developing cancer, there are things we can control (like lifestyle choices), and there are things we cannot control (like age and heredity). Some known risk factors include:

20

- Old age
- Family history of cancer
- Tobacco use
- Excessive alcohol consumption

25

- Obesity
- Poor dietary choices
- Excessive exposure to UV light
- Exposure to occupational chemicals and radiation

Cancer symptoms can vary widely depending on which organ is affected and how far the cancer has spread (**stage**). Some general symptoms include excessive fatigue; unexplained weight loss; poor appetite or difficulty eating; swollen lymph nodes; skin changes; and night sweats. Advanced cancers can cause **persistent** bleeding from the affected body part, such as the lungs or colon. Diagnosis is typically made through a combination of blood tests, imaging (including CT and MRI scans), and a **biopsy** of affected tissue. Once the doctor, usually an oncologist, has made a diagnosis, he or she will discuss a treatment plan with the patient. There are more than 200 types and subtypes of cancer, with a variety of treatments and therapies depending on the type and stage of cancer. Treatments might include chemotherapy, surgery, or focused radiation. Use of newer experimental therapies might involve enrolling patients into clinical trials.

30

35

In Japan, the mortality from cancer has steadily increased over the years. For men, the leading cause of death was from lung cancer, followed by stomach cancer, and colorectal

40

cancer. In women, the leading cause of death was from colorectal cancer followed by lung cancer. It is interesting to note that studies in Japan have stated 50% of cancers are preventable and related to lifestyle (such as with smoking).

◐ Words and Phrases

non-communicable 非伝染性の	stage ステージ、段階、時期
mutation 突然変異	persistent 長引く、執拗に続く
genes 遺伝子	biopsy 生体組織検査、生検
pollutants 汚染物質	

Language Point   **Affect vs Effect**

Affect and Effect are commonly mistaken. Both can be verbs and nouns, but Affect is more commonly used as verb while Effect is more often a noun.

Health is affected by lifestyle choices.
The effect was felt nationwide.

G Research #2 – Anatomy

a) Work alone. Label 6 common symptoms of lung cancer. If you do NOT know an answer, leave it blank.
    NOTE In part (a) do NOT look online for the answers.
b) After, work with a partner and discuss your answers. Fill in any of the answers you are missing.
c) Next, work with your partner and check your answers online.
d) Finally, your teacher will give you the answers. Check to see if your answers are correct.

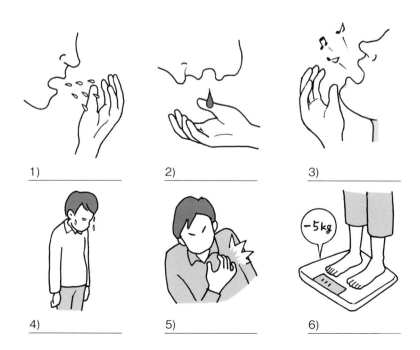

1) _____   2) _____   3) _____

4) _____   5) _____   6) _____

Make a team of 3-4 members. Choose one type of cancer from the box below and research the two following points. After each team is finished, share your answers.

Common Types of Cancer (choose one):

☐ breast cancer ☐ colorectal cancer

☐ lung cancer ☐ pancreatic cancer

☐ stomach cancer ☐ kidney cancer

☐ leukemia ☐ prostate cancer

Signs/Symptoms:

_____

_____

Treatment:

_____

_____

EXTENSIONS ➡ What are the 4 stages of cancer? Draw a chart and include the signs / symptoms at each stage.

_____

_____

Some say that the risk of some forms of cancer can be reduced or prevented by changing our lifestyle habits. What do you think? What ways can you lower your risk of cancer?

a) Work with a team of 3-4 members. Research and discuss 5 ways to lower the risk of cancer. Be ready to give reasons for your choices.

5 Ways to Lower the Risk of Cancer
1)
2)
3)
4)
5)

b) After presenting, discuss which team has the most effective list and why.

Project – Lifestyle Questionnaire

a) Work with a team of 3-4 members.
b) Create a set of questions about lifestyle habits in regard to preventable cancer. You can use the ideas from the discussion in Section I.
c) Interview your classmates and collect their answers.
d) What areas do students need to adjust to help reduce their risk? What areas do they NOT need to adjust?
e) Share the data from your survey on a poster with the class.

 Presentation Skills – Using Images in Your Presentation

Images are important in your presentation to convey meaning. However, presenters can make errors in selecting the right kind of images and have presentations that look unprofessional. Below is some advice for correctly using images:

1) Don't use blurry or low resolution, pixelated pictures. Look for photos that are high quality. (Remember that pictures that look clear on small screen (like your smartphone) might be blurry when enlarged or viewed on a larger screen or on a poster.)
2) Don't use watermarked photos. It looks unprofessional.
3) Don't stretch an image to fit on your slide. Crop the photo so it looks natural.
4) Don't use busy backgrounds or, with PPT, excessive animations. These things will distract the audience. Keep things simple to maximize the impact of your message.
5) Don't add too many images to a PPT slide or poster. With PPT, limit a slide to 2-4 images, or choose 1 image that sums up what you want to say.
6) Avoid silly or cartoonish clipart that can make your presentation look unprofessional. Use icons that are modern and more universally appealing.

EXTENSIONS ➡

a) Work with the same team members from Section J.
b) Put your team's poster on the wall.
c) Were there any problems with the use of images? What could be done to correct the problem(s)?

Reflection

Work alone. Think back over what you have learned in this unit and record your answers below.

1) What are some interesting things you have learned in this unit?
2) What do you want to improve about your learning?
3) If you did a presentation, what went well? What did not?

(A) What Do You Know?

What do you know about stress? Write 3 ideas below.

1) _____

_____

2) _____

_____

3) _____

_____

(B) Pair and Share #1

Talk with a partner and share your ideas from Section A. Remember to ask follow-up questions or make comments as your partner shares their answers:

- I wrote down _____. What did you write?
- What else did you write about?
- Yeah, same here! / That's what I think!
- Great answers! Here are some of mine.

(C) Paired Listening

011
1-11

a) Work with a partner. Listen to a podcast about stress. Take notes as you listen and answer the questions below.

1) What is *karoshi*?
2) What was number 4 in the Top 5 countdown for managing stress?
3) What are the benefits of number 4?
4) What is next week's topic?

b) Work with a partner and check your answers.

EXTENSIONS → What is "work-life balance"? Research online and find countries with a good work-life balance and countries with a poor one.

_____

_____

D Research #1 – Managing Stress

Everyone has stress. How you manage it on a daily basis is important. What are some ways to manage or reduce stress? Research online and list 10 methods of managing or reducing stress.

What Are 10 Ways to Manage or Reduce Stress?
1)
2)
3)
4)
5)
6)
7)
8)
9)
10)

E Pair and Share #2

Compare your answers from Section D with a classmate. Which answers are the same? Which answers are different? Discuss and decide which method is the most interesting on each of your lists. Give reasons to support your thinking.

A: Which method did you find the most interesting?

B: I thought making time for hobbies was interesting. I think that this is a great way to reduce stress. How about you?

EXTENSIONS ➡ Which of the methods from your list do you think is the least effective? Why?

Ⓕ Reading – Stress

Everyone experiences stress in their life. Stress is the body and brain's reaction to life's challenges and demands. These challenges and demands (or **stressors**) come in different shapes and sizes. Stressors might be something new or unexpected, or even something that is dangerous. Your body is designed to react and protect you against these different stressors. It
5 is important to note that in some situations stress can have a positive effect, helping you stay motivated, alert, energetic, or helping you avoid danger. Simply stated, stress can help you meet the challenges of life. This might include learning to drive, doing a presentation in front of a large audience, or hitting a homerun at a baseball game. However, what about the other kinds of stress that may have a negative effect on the body?

10 There are two basic types of stress: one is **acute** and the other is **chronic**. Acute stress happens to everyone from time to time. This type of stress tends to be caused by a short-termed challenge or one-off event, and afterward we recover from it. Acute stressors can range from being surprised by the sound of thunder, having a job interview, riding on a roller coaster, or losing your smartphone. In contrast, chronic stress happens over a long period of
15 time (weeks, months, or years) and results from problems that do not seem to go away. With chronic stress, there is little or no chance to relax. Some chronic stress may be external (being bullied at work or school, a problem in the family, or having a loud next-door neighbor), while others may be internal (**perfectionism**, **pessimistic** thinking, and/or lack of flexibility).

Chronic stress can affect both the mind and the body and varies from one person to the
20 next. Symptoms may include:

- Aches and pains
- A lack of energy or insomnia
- Headaches and dizziness
- Chest pain
25 - High blood pressure

- Digestive issues
- Lack of sexual interest
- Thinking and memory problems
- Skin conditions
- Depression and anxiety

Over time, chronic stress can have a serious effect on you physically and mentally. Conditions like heart disease, high blood pressure, depression, addiction disorders, and ulcers are just a few of the impacts that stress can have on your body. One example of chronic stress is *karoshi* (death from overwork). In a **workaholic** society, *karoshi* can have a serious
30 impact on a person's life. A study stated that, "In 2020, the number of people committing suicide due to problems related to their working situation reached 1,918 in Japan. The death numbers peaked in 2011 with almost 2,700 suicide victims in total."

How to best manage chronic stress varies from person to person, but the first step is to recognize one's stressors. Sometimes a mental health professional (psychiatrist, psychologist,
35 counselor, or health and wellness coach) can be helpful for this. Treatments target the

individual's specific symptoms and may include things like **behavior therapy**, medication, a change in diet, or increased exercise. What is important is to seek a healthcare professional if you need help or advice.

Words and Phrases

stressors ストレス要因、有害因子
acute （病気が）急性の
chronic （病気が）慢性の
perfectionism 完全主義

pessimistic 悲観的な、悲観主義の
workaholic ワーカホリック、仕事中毒の人
behavior therapy 行動療法

Language Point — **Uncountable Nouns**

Some nouns in English are uncountable and do not take "S":

- advice
- stuff

- work
- homework

- high blood pressure
- thunder

G **Research #2 – Anatomy**

a) Work alone. What are the headings for the diagram below? Read the symptoms and conditions under each box numbered 1-7. Think about what system or body part matches the symptoms or conditions. If you do NOT know an answer, leave it blank. NOTE In part (a) do NOT look online for the answers.

b) After, work with a partner and discuss your answers. Fill in any of the answers you are missing.

c) Next, work with your partner and check your answers online.

d) Finally, your teacher will give you the answers. Check to see if your answers are correct.

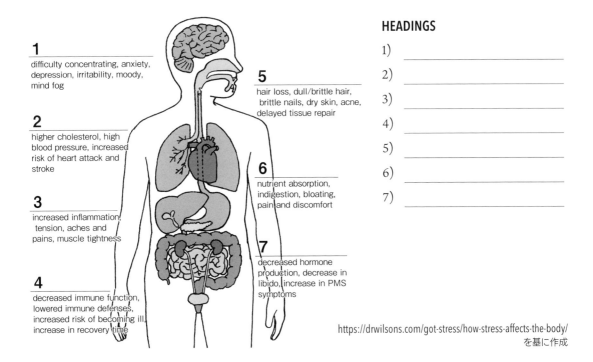

1 _____
difficulty concentrating, anxiety, depression, irritability, moody, mind fog

2 _____
higher cholesterol, high blood pressure, increased risk of heart attack and stroke

3 _____
increased inflammation, tension, aches and pains, muscle tightness

4 _____
decreased immune function, lowered immune defenses, increased risk of becoming ill, increase in recovery time

5 _____
hair loss, dull/brittle hair, brittle nails, dry skin, acne, delayed tissue repair

6 _____
nutrient absorption, indigestion, bloating, pain and discomfort

7 _____
decreased hormone production, decrease in libido, increase in PMS symptoms

HEADINGS

1) _____
2) _____
3) _____
4) _____
5) _____
6) _____
7) _____

https://drwilsons.com/got-stress/how-stress-affects-the-body/
を基に作成

H Research #3 – Group Work

Make a team of 3-4 members. Choose one of the headings from Section G and research more about how the heading is impacted by stress. When researching, think about problems with a person's body, mind, and behavior. After each team is finished, share your answers.

Heading: _____

Body	Mind	Behavior

EXTENSIONS ➡ A phobia is an unrealistic fear of an object or situation. Research online about one kind of phobia that you find interesting. What kind of phobia is it? What are the symptoms? Are there any treatments?

_____

_____

I Discussion – Childhood Stress: Is it Positive or Negative?

Positive stress in childhood might make us stronger as adults. However, some kinds of negative stress could also cause problems later on like mental illness or depression. What is your opinion about childhood stress? Is it mostly positive or is it mostly negative?

Work with a team of 3-4 members. Discuss the good points about childhood stress and the bad points. After discussing in your team, vote whether childhood stress is mostly positive or mostly negative. Be ready to give reasons for your choice.

Good Points	Bad Points

J Project – Advice

a) Work with a team of 3-4 members. List one way school life can cause you negative stress. After, research and brainstorm some ways to manage and reduce that stress. Remember to consider body, mind, and behavior.

Stress	Body	Mind	Behavior
Advice			

b) Create a team poster and share your team's information from Part J.

K Presentation Skills – References and Citations

Plagiarism is very serious. Plagiarism is when someone copies information as one's own, without citing and referencing the original creator. Whether it is a presentation, an essay, or an academic paper, you must cite the appropriate outside source(s) for any idea not your own. Below is some advice on how to include citations and references for presentations:

1) With PPT or posters, you can use in-text citations showing the author and date (Yamanaka, S. 2012), much like in some academic papers.
2) Be sure to cite particular facts (like data, charts, or tables).
3) You should cite images or clip art if they are not your own or available as "free share."
4) List all your references at the end of your PPT or poster. With PPT, add a second reference slide for photo credits or image sources.
5) There are several different formats (AMA, APA, MLA, Chicago, etc.) for citations and references. Be sure to check the format that you will need for your presentation. If no specific guidance is given, choose a format and BE CONSISTENT!

EXTENSIONS

a) Work with the same team members from Section J.
b) Choose one of the formats listed in Section K number 5.
c) Check your search history on your device to find the websites you used in Section J.
d) Add the in-text citations and references to your work in Section J.
e) Share your answers with other teams.

L Reflection

Work alone. Think back over what you have learned in this unit and record your answers below.

1) What are some interesting things you have learned in this unit?
2) What do you want to improve about your learning?
3) If you did a presentation, what went well? What did not?

Sleep

Ⓐ What Do You Know?

Why do you think sleep is important? Write 3 ideas below.

1) _____

_____

2) _____

_____

3) _____

_____

_____

Ⓑ Pair and Share #1

Talk with a partner and share your ideas from Section A. Remember to ask follow-up questions or make comments as your partner shares their answers:

- I've heard about…
- I've heard about that too.
- That's something I'm also interested in.
- What was one of your ideas?

Ⓒ Paired Listening

a) Work with a partner. Listen to the conversation between two friends. Take notes as you listen and answer the questions below.

1) What did Steve dream of?
2) When did the Aberfan disaster happen?
3) How many children died?
4) What part of the brain is mentioned in the dialogue?

b) Work with a partner and check your answers.

EXTENSIONS ➡ Do you think it is possible dreams could be premonitions? Have you ever had a vivid dream? Describe it to your partner.

_____

_____

D Research #1 – Sleep's Benefits and Consequences

Sleep is crucial to maintaining a healthy life. In fact you are more likely to die more quickly from sleep deprivation than food deprivation. A good night's sleep is considered to be a healthy 7-8 hours. What are the benefits of sleep and what are some of the consequences of a lack of sleep? Research online and make a list below.

Benefits of Good Sleep	Consequences of Poor Sleep
1)	1)
2)	2)
3)	3)
4)	4)
5)	5)
6)	6)
7)	7)
8)	8)
9)	9)
10)	10)

E Pair and Share #2

Compare your answers from Section D with a classmate. Which answers are the same? Which answers are different? Which of the above benefits is the most important? Have you ever experienced any negative effects due to sleep problems? Give reasons to support your thinking.

A: I think the greatest benefit of good sleep is that you can improve your memory. However, once I drank three energy drinks every night during my exam week, so I could stay awake and study more.

B: Me, too. Did it help with your memory?

EXTENSIONS ➡ What are some helpful ways to get to sleep? What would you suggest if a friend was struggling with irregular sleep?

The average lifespan of a human is 79 years. Of those 79 years, humans spend a large portion of that time, an impressive 26 years, asleep. In fact, a further 7 years are spent trying to get to sleep! That's a massive total of 33 years in bed.

Much like recharging a smartphone, sleep is essential for recharging the body and mind each night. Yet many people regard sleep as time wasted and neglect to get the right amount that is believed to be healthy. A good eight hours every night is generally considered a healthy amount, with the elements of duration (how long), continuity (without interruption), and depth (a deep restorative sleep) all being achieved.

However, it is estimated that between 30%-45% of the world's adult population have sleep problems, threatening the health and quality of many lives, and qualifying it as a global **epidemic**. The human body has four biological rhythms, called **circadian rhythms**. These circadian rhythms are synchronized with the brain's "master clock," located in the **pineal gland**, and are directly influenced by environmental cues such as sunlight. The circadian rhythm involved in the sleep-wake cycle is particularly affected by light and darkness. If this circadian rhythm is properly aligned with day and night, it is more likely that a good sleep will occur.

A good sleep can be characterized into two distinctly different phases that alternate periodically throughout the night: They are non-rapid eye movement (**NREM**) and rapid eye movement (**REM**). NREM is further divided into three stages. Stage 1 is often referred to as relaxed wakefulness. If woken from this state, it is quite common for people to believe they had not fallen asleep at all. Stage 2 is characterized by a lack of eye movement, and dreaming during this time is rare. Stage 3 is known as deep sleep or slow wave sleep. In this stage, a particular type of low frequency brain wave, called a delta wave, takes over and dominates brain activity. Brain waves are rhythmic repetitive patterns of **neural** activity in the central nervous system and can be recorded on an electroencephalogram (**EEG**). Some dreaming can occur, but it is not as common as in REM sleep. During these stages of NREM, the body replenishes its energy and repairs cells, tissues, and muscles. It also strengthens the body's immune system. NREM sleep is followed by REM sleep, in which we dream.

In a healthy eight hours of sleep, the brain goes into REM about four times (cycles). The times in which we are in REM can range from only ten minutes in the first cycle to an hour in the fourth cycle. REM is characterized by rapid eye movement, fast and irregular breathing, as well as an increased heart rate and brain activity similar to being awake. During REM, a temporary **paralysis** can be experienced as the brain signals the spinal cord to **inhibit** arm and leg movement. Due to the increase in brain activity, this is the state in which **vivid** dreams may occur. REM sleep is thought to be beneficial to learning, mood, and memory.

Words and Phrases

epidemic 伝染性の、流行性の	neural 神経（系）の
circadian rhythms 概日リズム、生物リズム	EEG 脳波図、脳波計
pineal gland 松果体	paralysis 麻痺
NREM ノンレム	inhibit/inhibitions （活動・興奮の）抑制
REM レム、急速眼球運動	vivid はっきりとした、活発な

Language Point   -ed vs -ing

Adjectives with -ed or -ing endings are sometimes easy to confuse. Generally, -ed is used for people and animals, and -ing is used for situations and objects.

I was <u>bored</u> last night.
That movie is pretty <u>boring</u>.

G Research #2 – Anatomy

a) Work alone. What problems due to lack of sleep might occur in the areas of the body indicated below? If you do NOT know an answer, leave it blank. NOTE In part (a) do NOT look online for the answers.

b) After, work with a partner and discuss your answers. Fill in any of the answers you are missing.

c) Next, work with your partner and check your answers online.

d) Finally, your teacher will give you the answers. Check to see if your answers are correct.

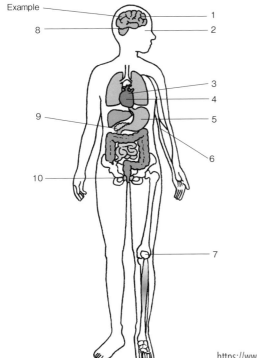

(Example) memory issues

1) _____

2) _____

3) _____

4) _____

5) _____

6) _____

7) _____

8) _____

9) _____

10) _____

https://www.healthline.com/health/sleep-deprivation/effects-on-body を基に作成

H Research #3 – Group Work

Make a team of 3-4 members. Choose one problem from Section G and further research the topic as it relates to sleep. After each team is finished, share your answers.

Problem: _____

What are the effects?

_____

_____

EXTENSIONS ➡ How does the use of a smartphone before bed affect a person's sleep? Do you have any advice to help smartphone users have a better night's sleep?

_____

_____

I Discussion – Are Sleeping Problems a Modern Phenomenon?

Given that so many people suffer from sleep-related problems, is this due to a modern lifestyle? Is our chance of getting enough of a healthy sleep deteriorating? Did our ancestors have problems with sleeping?

Work with a team of 3-4 members. Think about whether sleep-related problems are a modern phenomenon or not. Try to come up with good points and bad points about our modern lifestyle relating to having a healthy night's sleep.

Good Points	Bad Points

J Project – Sleep Disorders and Related Illnesses

a) Work with a team of 3-4 members. Choose one kind of problem from the list below:

☐ insomnia ☐ obstructive sleep apnea ☐ central sleep apnea ☐ restless leg syndrome
☐ narcolepsy ☐ parasomnias ☐ REM sleep behavior disorder
☐ non-24-hour sleep-wake disorder ☐ excessive daytime sleepiness

b) Create a team poster to share what you learned. Include the following information on your poster:

- What are the causes?
- What are the symptoms or consequences?
- What are the treatments/are there any treatments?
- How can we prevent it?
- When should we talk to a doctor?
- Who is likely to suffer from it?
- Include photos, illustrations, and/or diagrams to support your research.
- Include references, showing where you found the information online.

K Presentation Skills – Presentation Practice

You should always be well-prepared for any presentation you will give. In the extra time before making your presentation, PRACTICE! It will help you relax and be more confident and make you look more professional. Below are some guidelines for practicing before your big day:

1) Rehearse in front of family or friends. This will give you a chance to work on eye contact, body language, and voice inflection. An audience can also give you feedback about the points you need to work on.
2) If you don't have an audience, simply practice out loud. You can speak in front of a mirror or you can videotape yourself presenting. You can watch the video afterward and find your weak points.
3) Be sure to stand up when you practice. There is a big difference in your energy when you are sitting vs standing while presenting. Also, when you present in front of an audience, you will most likely be standing.
4) Practice more than once! Some presenters say you should practice ten times to perfect all the elements of your presentation.
5) Time yourself. Most presentations have a time limit. Afterward, check your content. If you are rushed for time, are there any areas you can cut? If you have too much time, is there any content you can expand?
6) Plan where you will place pauses or slow down your speech. Pausing before a key point can have a powerful effect in your presentation.
7) Watch videos of other speakers online and use their skills when you present.

EXTENSIONS

a) Work with the same team members from Section J.
b) Read the mini-speech your teacher gives to your team.
c) Individuals take turns standing and sharing the speech.
d) Team members in the audience: Give both positive and constructive feedback.
e) When one speaker finishes, select a new speaker and repeat.
f) After all members are finished, repeat sharing the speech a second time. Did you improve?

L Reflection

Work alone. Think back over what you have learned in this unit and record your answers below.

1) What are some interesting things you have learned in this unit?
2) What do you want to improve about your learning?
3) If you did a presentation, what went well? What did not?

Unit 8 Addiction

A What Do You Know?

What do you know about addiction? Write 3 ideas below.

1) _____

_____

2) _____

_____

3) _____

_____

B Pair and Share #1

Talk with a partner and share your ideas from Section A. Remember to ask follow-up questions or make comments as your partner shares their answers:

- It's interesting that you included...!
- Why is that?/How is that?
- I thought the same!/I would have thought differently.
- Is that true? I never knew that./I would never have included that.

C Paired Listening

a) Work with a partner. Listen to two friends, Chas and Marty, talk about addiction. Take notes as you listen and answer the questions below.

1) What does Chas say Marty is addicted to?
2) What is dopamine?
3) What does Chas admit to being addicted to?

b) Work with a partner and check your answers.

EXTENSIONS ➡ Do you think you are addicted to using your smartphone? In what ways?

_____

_____

D   Research #1 – Addictive Drugs

There are many drugs available to us today. Many of these drugs are legal, but there are also a large number of drugs that are illegal. The addicitive potential of drugs ranges widely, from mild to dangerous. Research about drugs, their effects, and the ways that they may be addictive. Remember: Just because a drug is legal does not mean it is not addictive.

Drug's Name	Effects/How It Is Addictive

E   Pair and Share #2

Compare your answers from Section D with a classmate. Which answers are the same? Which answers are different? Discuss and decide which drug is the MOST addictive/dangerous on your lists. Give reasons to support your thinking.

A: I think heroin is the most addictive and dangerous drug because so many people say once they try it, they can't stop. Also, many people have died from it.

B: I don't think heroin is the most dangerous addicitve drug. Many more people have died from tobacco.

EXTENSIONS ➡ What do you think is the most addictive drug in Japan? Why?

_____

_____

F Reading – Addiction

Rather than simply a personal choice, addiction is now widely accepted to be a **chronic** medical disease. Addiction is considered a disease because it alters the way the brain functions, just as cardiovascular disease effects the way the heart functions. Addiction generally occurs through the regular use of **substances** or a repeated behavior that becomes **compulsive**, 5 regardless of any possible harmful consequences.

Perhaps the most commonly known and most serious type of addiction is the addiction to drugs and alcohol. Drug and alcohol addiction is often considered more serious as its effects, in many cases, may be easier to identify. However, there are a number of other addictions, all of which can negatively impact lives, sometimes with devastating 10 consequences. Examples of other addictions are gambling, **binge** eating disorder (food addiction), shopping addiction, and more recently, internet addiction.

What all these addictions have in common is how the brain, or particular areas of the brain, react and behave when presented with certain substances or situations. When addicted, the brain develops what is known as **incentive salience**. Incentive salience is a process in the 15 brain in which desire and reward become the primary motivation. This **cognitive process** is regulated by a **neurotransmitter** called **dopamine**.

Many types of drugs can cause a big increase in dopamine. These dopamine molecules are "chemical messages" between neurons in the brain, and produce a feeling of satisfaction in your natural reward system. In other words, the addictive behavior makes a person feel 20 good. In the case of addictive drugs, with regular use, the dose might need to be increased to achieve the same "reward feeling." Over time, the brain's ability to naturally produce dopamine **deteriorates**, giving the user a sense of **dependency** on the particular drug to regenerate the dopamine that is otherwise absent.

With the absence of natural dopamine, a regular drug user will feel low and want to feel 25 better. When this occurs, incentive salience can result in the constant craving of addiction. In other words, the user needs to take more of the drug just to feel normal. Symptoms of addiction are variable and can range from mild to life-threatening.

Words and Phrases

chronic （病気が）慢性の	cognitive process 認知プロセス
substance 物質、薬物	neurotransmitter 神経伝達物質
compulsive 衝動強迫的な	dopamine ドーパミン
binge 過度にすること、飲み（食べ）過ぎる	deteriorate 低下する、悪化する
incentive salience インセンティブ・サリエンス	dependency 依存

The Use of "the" with Body Organs

Often the definite article "the" is used with organs and organ systems. It is used even with an initial mention. Since there is only one brain, the definite article is required.

What all these addictions have in common is how the brain, or particular areas of the brain, react and behave when presented with certain substances or situations.

Ⓖ Research #2 – Anatomy

a) Work alone. Try to fill in the blanks, identifying which organs can be impacted by long-term alcohol use. If you do NOT know an answer, leave it blank. NOTE In part (a) do NOT look online for the answers.

b) After, work with a partner and discuss your answers. Fill in any of the answers you are missing.

c) Next, work with your partner and check your answers online.

d) Finally, your teacher will give you the answers. Check to see if your answers are correct.

1) _____
2) _____
3) _____
4) _____
5) _____
6) _____
7) _____

Ⓗ Research #3 – Group Work

Make a team of 3-4 members. Research the function of one of the organs from Section G. Also, research how this organ is affected in regard to chronic alcohol use. After each team is finished, share your answers.

Organ's name: _____
Important functions:

_____

How it is affected by chronic alcohol use:

_____

EXTENSIONS ➡ Alcohol-related Liver Disease (ARLD) is the most common disease suffered by alcoholics. What is ARLD? What are the symptoms? What is the treatment? Research online and find the answers.

_____

_____

Ⓘ Discussion – Should Smoking Be Banned?

A number of countries around the world have successfully reduced tobacco consumption through various campaigns and restrictions. To protect the next generation, New Zealand has gone further, becoming the first country to make smoking illegal by 2025. Though the number of smokers may have decreased globally (from 21% in 2005 to 19% as of 2021), in countries such as China, the number of people who regularly smoke is increasing and is believed to be as many as 300 million. What is your opinion on smoking? Should it be banned completely or are there any social reasons why it should remain legal?

Work with a team of 3-4 members. Discuss the reasons, for and against, on whether smoking should remain legal or should become illegal. After discussing, take a group vote whether it should be banned or not. NOTE Be ready to give reasons for your choice!

Reasons Why Smoking Should Remain Legal	Reasons Why Smoking Should Become Banned

Ⓙ Project – Types of Addiction

a) Work with a team of 3-4 members. Choose one kind of addiction from the list below and research about it:

☐ gambling addiction   ☐ alcoholism   ☐ opioid addiction
☐ smoking (nicotine) addiction   ☐ internet/smartphone addiction
☐ shopping addiction   ☐ adrenaline addiction
☐ binge eating/food addiction   ☐ addiction to sleeping pills   ☐ cocaine addiction
☐ methamphetamine ("crystal meth," "ice," or "shabu") addiction

b) Create a warning PPT to share what you learned. Include the following information on your PPT:

- What kind of addiction is it?   • How can the addiction be defined/diagnosed?
- What are the physical symptoms of the addiction?
- How does it impact a person's life or the lives of those around them?
- Include photos, illustrations, and/or diagrams to support your research.
- Include references, showing where you found the information online.

Presentation Skills – Do's and Don'ts of PowerPoint Presentations

PowerPoint (PPT) is a quick and easy way to organize ideas and information for presentations. Below is advice to help you improve your PPT presentations.

Do

1. **Be consistent**

   Design a simple template. Be consistent with elements such as fonts, colors, and background.

2. **Organize your information clearly**

   Be brief and clear. Avoid crowding your slides with information. Aim for no more than 3-8 sentences/phrases per slide. If you are using lists, set a limit of 6 points per slide. Also, use good quality images that complement your ideas.

3. **End with a summary slide or a "take home message"**

   Go through your key points or arguments by including a summary slide at the end of your presentation. The most important sections of a presentation are the beginning and end. The beginning is the main opportunity to catch the attention of the audience, and a summary slide helps ensure that the audience understands the key information.

   Another way to end your presentation is with a "take home message," where you share one or two key points from your talk that are easy for the audience to understand. You can also suggest the audience to take action. This is an effective way to help the audience remember your talk.

Don't

1. **Put too much information on one slide**

   Write only the most important information on each slide.

2. **Just read the slides**

   The slides should feature only the essence of your message. Know your topic well and tell your audience about the finer details during the presentation.

3. **Rush**

   Give your audience time to read each slide. When opening a new slide, give the audience a little time to read the slide before you start talking.

EXTENSIONS ➡

a) Work with the same team members from Section J.
b) Review the list of Do's and Don'ts of PowerPoint.
c) Open the PowerPoint link: https://www.alzheimersresearchuk.org/wp-content/uploads/2020/03/Researcher-Toolkit-Presentation.pptx
d) As a group, quickly read the PPT.
e) Did the PPT follow the points of the Do's and Don'ts list? Discuss with your group.

L **Reflection**

Work alone. Think back over what you have learned in this unit and record your answers below.

1) What are some interesting things you have learned in this unit?
2) What do you want to improve about your learning?
3) If you did a presentation, what went well? What did not?

Alzheimer's Disease and Dementia

A What Do You Know?

What do you know about Alzheimer's disease and dementia? Write 3 ideas below.

1) _____

_____

2) _____

_____

3) _____

_____

B Pair and Share #1

Talk with a partner and share your ideas from Section A. Remember to ask follow-up questions or make comments as your partner shares their answers:

- That's interesting!
- Sorry, I didn't catch that last part.
- You probably heard that...
- Oh, I almost forgot to mention...

C Paired Listening

017
2-3

a) Work with a partner. Listen to a classroom teacher talk about Alzheimer's disease and dementia. Take notes as you listen and answer the questions below.

1) What are the symptoms of Alzheimer's disease?
2) What kind of memories are usually lost first?

b) Work with a partner and check your answers.

EXTENSIONS ➡ Do you have a good memory? What can people do to improve their memory?

_____

_____

When the brain is damaged, it can affect many different things, including memory, movement, and even a person's personality. Think of 10 illnesses that can damage the brain. Research online and make a list below. Do NOT forget to include signs and symptoms for each illness.

Brain Illnesses	Signs/Symptoms
1)	
2)	
3)	
4)	
5)	
6)	
7)	
8)	
9)	
10)	

E Pair and Share #2

Compare your answers from Section D with a classmate. Which answers are the same? Which answers are different? Discuss and decide which brain illness is the most common. Give reasons to support your thinking.

A: I think dementia is the most common because there is a high chance that elderly people will get it.

B: I have a different opinion. I chose depression. From the research I did online, I found that more than 264 million people suffer from depression worldwide.

EXTENSIONS ➡ What do you think is the most common brain illness amongst young people? Why?

_____

_____

F Reading – Alzheimer's Disease and Dementia

Research has shown that the causes of dementia are complex, and unfortunately there is no certain way to prevent it. While age is the biggest risk factor for dementia, our genetics and our lifestyle also appear to play a role. There may not be much we can do about our genetics, but we have a lot more control over our daily habits and behaviours. What lifestyle choices
5　can we make to help prevent dementia?

Keeping your mind active is likely to reduce your risk of dementia. Regularly challenging yourself mentally seems to build up the brain's ability to cope with disease. Find something you enjoy doing that challenges your brain and do it regularly. It is important to find something that you can maintain. For example, study for a qualification or course, learn a new language,
10　do puzzles, crosswords or quizzes, or read challenging books.

Evidence suggests that physical exercise may improve **cognition** not only in older adults with normal **cognitive function**, but also in people who have trouble remembering and making decisions that affect everyday life. The Mental Activity and eXercise (MAX) trial tested the usefulness of combining physical exercise and brain training in adults suffering
15　from memory loss. The **participants** in the study did some form of exercise for 60 minutes a day, 3 days a week. After 12 weeks, all the participant groups showed stronger memory skills. The study found that the amount of activity is more important than the type of activity. Therefore, why not make more time for the types of exercise that you enjoy?

Nutrition also has a role in preventing cognitive decline and dementia. The Mediterranean
20　diet is high in vegetables, fruits, legumes, fish, and unsaturated fats such as olive oil. A recent review that included 18 studies, 5 of which were **randomized control trials (RCTs)**, showed that the Mediterranean diet helps delay cognitive decline by improving memory and language skills. The diet was also found to have a positive effect on **executive functioning** skills, the mental processes that enable us to plan, focus attention, remember instructions, and juggle
25　multiple tasks successfully. In another study, the American Academy of **Neurology** reported that participants who followed the diet closely performed better on cognitive tests and showed less **brain** volume **shrinkage** and fewer **protein biomarkers** associated with Alzheimer's disease. For a healthier brain, some experts suggest eating fish at least twice a week and regularly enjoying healthy salads drizzled in olive oil.

30　While there is not one single way to prevent dementia, maintaining a healthy diet and exercising both mind and body can help people reduce their risk of the condition.

📝 **Words and Phrases**

cognition/cognitive function 認知／認知的機能　　neurology 神経学
participant 研究協力者　　　　　　　　　　　　 brain shrinkage 脳の萎縮
randomized control trials (RCTs) 無作為化比較試験　protein biomarkers タンパク質バイオマーカー
executive functioning 遂行機能

An abbreviation is a shortened form of a written word or phrase. Abbreviations may be used to save space and time, and to avoid the repetition of long words and phrases.

- Doctor (Dr.) • Mental Activity and eXercise trial (MAX)

Acronyms are a type of abbreviation, and are usually made up of the initial letters of a phrase.

- randomized control trial (RCT) • blood pressure (BP)

G Research #2 – Anatomy

a) Work alone. Label the parts of the brain below. If you do NOT know an answer, leave it blank.
   NOTE In part (a) do NOT look online for the answers.
b) After, work with a partner and discuss your answers. Fill in any of the answers you are missing.
c) Next, work with your partner and check your answers online.
d) Your teacher will give you the answers. Check to see if your answers are correct.

1) _____
2) _____
3) _____
4) _____
5) _____
6) _____

H Research #3 – Group Work

Make a team of 3-4 members. Choose one area of the brain from Section G and research its functions. After each team is finished, share your answers.

Area's name: _____
Important functions: _____
_____
_____

EXTENSIONS ➡ Which area of the brain is the most vital for survival? What are its functions? Research online and find the answers.

Discussion – Is It Better for People With Advanced Alzheimer's or Dementia to Live with Their Families or in Care Homes?

A person with Alzheimer's or dementia will need more care and support as their condition progresses. What is your opinion: Should people with dementia or advanced Alzheimer's live in care homes or with their family until the end of their lives?

Work with a team of 3-4 members. Discuss the advantages and disadvantages of care homes and living with families for people with advanced Alzheimer's or dementia. After discussing, decide with your team which is the best place for people with advanced Alzheimer's or dementia: Care homes or living with families?

	Advantages	Disadvantages
Care Homes		
Living with Families		

J **Project – Activities for People with Alzheimer's or Dementia**

a) Work with a group of 3-4 members. Choose one of the activities from the list below and research about it:

☐ Tai Chi ☐ yoga ☐ walking group ☐ painting class ☐ drama group
☐ book club ☐ potluck party ☐ gardening ☐ spa treatment ☐ music therapy

b) Create a PPT to share what you have learned. Include the following information in your presentation:

- Introduce the activity.
- What are the general benefits of this activity?
- How could this activity benefit a person with Alzheimer's or dementia?
- How can the activity be modified to be more Alzheimer's or dementia-friendly?
- Include photos, illustrations, and/or diagrams to support your research.
- Include references, showing where you found the information online.

Presentation Skills – How to Write and Deliver a Hook

A presentation often begins with the speaker introducing themselves, and the subject they will speak about. This is all well and fine, but if the speaker is just one of many, and the audience is fatigued and ready to go home, the audience may not be paying full attention. This is where a hook is useful, immediately grabbing the audience's attention and allowing them to focus on you. So, what is a hook? A hook is like a topic sentence/story but designed to increase the attention of the audience. There are many types of hooks but here are 4 common examples. A hook can be:

1) A question
2) A little-known or surprising statistic
3) An interesting or funny anecdote
4) A shocking or surprising fact, action, or behavior (related to your topic!)

EXTENSIONS

a) Work with the same team members from Section J.
b) Choose one of the hooks from examples 1-4 above, and as a group practice writing a hook for your topic.
c) Perform your hook for the other teams.
d) Listeners: give feedback to the speaker.

Examples

Topic: music therapy

Hook 1: How many people worldwide like to listen to music each day?

Hook 2: There is research that shows that popular music can unlock memories.

Hook 3: I remember being at a party and hearing an old song from my childhood. Suddenly, I remembered being 10-years old.

Hook 4: About 6 million people in the US suffer from Alzheimer's. Music therapy is helping some of these people.

Hook Connectivity/Relevance Scoring Scale

Great	Good	Poor

Reflection

Work alone. Think back over what you have learned in this unit and record your answers below.

1) What are some interesting things you have learned in this unit?
2) What do you want to improve about your learning?
3) If you did a presentation, what went well? What did not?

Infectious Diseases

Ⓐ What Do You Know?

What do you know about infectious diseases? Write 3 ideas below.

1) _____

_____

2) _____

_____

3) _____

_____

Ⓑ Pair and Share #1

Share your ideas from Section A with a partner. Don't forget to ask follow-up questions or make comments as your partner shares their answers:

- Really? I didn't know that!
- Why did you write that down?
- Yes, that's (very) true.
- That makes sense.

Ⓒ Paired Listening

a) Work with a partner. Listen to two friends, Frances and Jiro, talk about infectious diseases. Take notes as you listen and answer the questions below.

1) Why does Frances think the tradition of *Shichi-Go-San* (Seven-Five-Three) started?
2) Does Jiro know why it started?
3) Where did Jiro visit in Australia?
4) What did Jiro notice in the cemetery?

b) Work with a partner and check your answers.

EXTENSIONS ➡ What is the infant mortality rate in Japan? Has it improved? What is the MMR vaccine?

_____

_____

D Research #1 – Common Infectious Diseases

It is not uncommon for infants and young children to catch infectious diseases. Adults are also susceptible. What are some common infectious diseases? Are these diseases caused by bacteria (B) or viruses (V)? Research online and make a list below.

Common Infectious Diseases	Caused by Bacteria (B) or Virus (V)
1)	
2)	
3)	
4)	
5)	
6)	
7)	
8)	
9)	
10)	

E Pair and Share #2

Compare your answers from Section D with a classmate. Which answers are the same? Which answers are different? Discuss and give reasons to support your thinking.

A: The first infectious disease I thought of was the common cold.

B: Is it caused by a bacteria or a virus?

EXTENSIONS ➡ Who is most at risk from bacterial and viral infectious diseases?

_____

_____

F Reading – Infectious Diseases

       In 2008, October 15th was designated as "National Hand Washing Day" in many countries as part of an international public health awareness campaign. Since the onset of the COVID-19 pandemic in late 2019, the simple act of hand washing has become more important than ever. Long ago, children were often instructed to "wash your hands like a doctor" by
5 parents who had likely lived through or heard about the dangers of infectious diseases like **polio** and **rubella**. We perhaps owe this advice to a 19th century Hungarian **obstetrician**

named Ignaz Semmelweis, who observed that maternal **mortality rates** were reduced when doctors washed their hands with chlorine. These days, no one would argue that people are living longer and healthier lives, not only because of improved **hygiene**, but also due to the availability of clean water, access to nutritious food, comfortable and safe housing, and good quality health care. In addition, through scientific advancement, we now know much more about bacteria and viruses and how the body responds to these infectious agents. In order to fully understand this, knowledge of the immune system is paramount.

The immune response is comprised of both structural and functional components. The structural aspect consists of the lymphatic system, which includes organs such as the spleen, thymus, tonsils, and lymph nodes, connected to one another by an intricate network of lymphatic vessels. Lymph, the liquid that helps carry immune cells, passes through these organs on its journey back to the venous circulation, picking up foreign particles along the way. Immune cells begin as stem cells and arise from the **bone marrow**. These cells **differentiate** into red and white blood cells. It is the white blood cells, also called **leukocytes**, which are the primary cells of the immune system that react to foreign invaders (antigens). Immune cells recognize antigens in a variety of ways after they break through the body's first lines of defense—the skin, the airways, and gastrointestinal (GI) tract.

Immune cells participate in the functional aspect of the immune system, comprised of two parts: fast-acting **innate immunity** and slower **adaptive immunity**. When an antigenic foreign substance is detected, **dendritic cells** and mast cells are the first responders of the innate system, followed shortly by macrophages (phagocytes) and neutrophils, which trap the invaders. Dendritic cells are the go-between, communicating with and presenting antigens to the adaptive system. The adaptive system is primarily comprised of T and B cells. There are four kinds of T cells (helper, cytotoxic, regulatory, and memory) and two kinds of B cells (plasma and memory). The B cells are responsible for creating antibodies. This interdependent relationship between innate and adaptive immunity is mimicked by vaccination and used to fight a wide variety of infectious diseases.

However, many infectious diseases have evolved to stay one step ahead of the human immune system. They are often highly contagious, spreading quickly and easily from person to person via exhaled or expelled droplets that can be present in contaminated air or surfaces. Most people will be familiar with colds, as well as accusations of, "you gave me YOUR cold". Influenza ("the flu"), infectious conjunctivitis ("pink eye"), and childhood diseases such as measles are some examples of highly infectious viral diseases. Prior to the outbreak of COVID-19, influenza killed 650,000 people in a bad year. In 2020, tuberculosis (TB), a bacterial infectious disease, killed 1.5 million people worldwide. Many of these diseases are zoonotic in origin, meaning that they have spread from animals to humans. Some examples of **zoonotic diseases** are COVID-19 and influenza A. With the destruction of habitats and deforestation, human and animal interaction is more frequent than ever before. Add global

45 travel—approximately 1.5 billion people travelled in 2019—and it is not difficult to imagine that infectious diseases can spread more readily around the world than in days gone by. While vaccinations, medications (antivirals and antibiotics), and diagnostic procedures advance rapidly in response to pandemics like COVID-19, they still take time to be developed and tested for **efficacy** and safety. In the meantime, a piece of good old advice on how to slow
50 down the spread of infectious diseases may very well be "wash your hands like a doctor!"

Words and Phrases

polio ポリオ
rubella 風疹、三日ばしか
obstetrician 産科医
mortality rate 死亡率
hygiene 衛生（状態）
bone marrow 骨髄
differentiate 分化する

leukocytes リンパ球
innate immunity 自然免疫
adaptive immunity 適応免疫
dendritic cells 樹状細胞
zoonotic disease 人獣共通感染症
efficacy （薬などの）有効性、効きめ

Language Point   Instructions for Taking Medicine

It is important to follow the instructions when taking medicine. Below are some examples in English:
- Take with meals (qAC)
- Take 2 times a day (BID) before breakfast/dinner
- Take on an empty stomach
- Take by mouth/orally (PO)
- Take 3 times a day (TID) with meals
- Take once daily (Qday) after lunch
- Avoid alcohol   • Take at bedtime (HS)
- Apply topically to affected area

G Research #2 – Anatomy

a) Work alone. Label the organs of the immune system. If you do NOT know an answer, leave it blank.
   NOTE In part (a) do NOT look online for the answers.
b) After, work with a partner and discuss your answers. Fill in any of the answers you are missing.
c) Next, work with your partner and check your answers online.
d) Finally, your teacher will give you the answers. Check to see if your answers are correct.

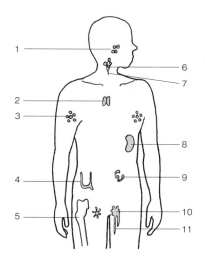

1) _____
2) _____
3) _____
4) _____
5) _____
6) _____
7) _____
8) _____
9) _____
10) _____
11) _____

H Research #3 – Group Work

Make a team of 3-4 members. Research the function of one of the organs in Section G. After each team is finished, share your answers.

Organ's Name	Location	Function

EXTENSIONS Tonsillitis is a common childhood disease. What is tonsillitis? What is the cause? What are the symptoms? What is the treatment? Research online and find the answers.

I Discussion – What Are the Three Worst Epidemics/Pandemics?

By definition, an epidemic is a disease that occurs at higher-than-expected rates within a local population, whereas a pandemic is worldwide. Both epidemics and pandemics have regularly occurred throughout our history. Some very serious ones date back hundreds or even thousands of years, while others have affected our modern world more recently.

a) Work with a team of 3-4 members. Research online and find the answers to the questions below. Also, be sure to take notes on the reasons for your choices.

- What is the worst epidemic/pandemic of the 21st century?
- What is worst epidemic/pandemic in Japan?
- What do you think is the worst epidemic/pandemic of all time?

b) Discuss with other teams. Which answers are similar? Which answers are different?

J Project – What Is the Difference Between a Common Cold and the Flu (Influenza)?

a) Work with a group of 3-4 members. Compare the causes, symptoms, and treatment of a common cold and the flu. Fill in the table below. Then research online and check if your ideas are correct.

	Causes	Symptoms	Treatment
Common Cold			
The Flu			

b) These days many healthcare clinics have visual display screens in waiting rooms showing information to help the public understand different illnesses. Use the information in part a) to create a PPT presentation that shows what you have learned. Your PPT should include the causes, symptoms, and treatment. In addition to this, think about photos, illustrations, or diagrams that could be used. Be sure to include references, showing where you found the information online.

K Presentation Skills – Giving Effective Conclusions

Did you know most people only remember the first and last things you tell them? Therefore, when it comes to giving a presentation, you definitely want people to remember your final words. Here are a few ways to effectively conclude a presentation.

Summarize: What do you want your audience to remember? Summarize and highlight again the key points of your presentation. This is a great way to ensure that your main points are appropriately communicated and that your audience is walking away with the information that you intended to convey. When summarizing the key points, give them context and show the audience exactly how they support your main argument.

Close Powerfully: Towards the end, it is time to choose your final words. The best option depends on the presenter, the topic, and the audience. One option is to end with a "call to action." Let the audience know what you want them to do next. Another effective strategy is to use a motivational quote; an inspirational quote can influence how audiences feel about a presentation overall. Or, end with a surprising statistic or information that will stick with the audience and encourage further thought on your topic. Depending on the subject matter, closing out a presentation with a joke can be a great way to drive a point home and leave your audience with something to remember.

Take Questions: At the end of your presentation, allow time to take any questions from the audience. A question and answer (Q&A) session gives the audience an opportunity to raise issues, helps keep engagement high, and allows you to further expand on your key points. Bring the Q&A session to a close, and offer to speak afterwards with audience members who did not have time to ask their questions.

EXTENSIONS
a) Work with the same members from Section J.
b) Review the tips for giving effective conclusions.
c) Open the link to watch a TED Talk on end-of-life care by BJ Miller. Skip ahead to the 14:35 mark to watch the end of the presentation. https://www.youtube.com/watch?v=apbSsILLh28
d) Did the presentation follow the advice for giving conclusions? Discuss with your group.

L Reflection

Work alone. Think back over what you have learned in this unit and record your answers below.

1) What are some interesting things you have learned in this unit?
2) What do you want to improve about your learning?
3) If you did a presentation, what went well? What did not?

HIV/AIDS and STDs

Ⓐ What Do You Know?

What do you know about HIV/AIDS and STDs (sexually transmitted diseases)? Write 3 ideas below.

1) _____

_____

2) _____

_____

3) _____

_____

Ⓑ Pair and Share #1

Share your ideas from Section A with a partner. Don't forget to ask follow-up questions or make comments as your partner shares their answers:

- Really?/No way!/I didn't know that.
- Is that so? I never heard that before!
- Really? I find that hard to believe.
- Oh really? I wrote some different ideas.

021 2-7 Ⓒ Paired Listening

a) Work with a partner. Listen to two friends, Jon and Yuki, talk about Dr. Yamanaka. Take notes as you listen and answer the questions below.

1) Where is the professor who won the Nobel Prize from?
2) Why are stem cells amazing?
3) What diseases are they talking about?
4) Why did Yuki say, "Oh no!"?

b) Work with a partner and check your answers.

EXTENSIONS ➡ What are some risk factors for getting HIV/AIDS and STDs?

_____

_____

Some commonly occurring STDs (sexually transmitted diseases) in Japan are the human papilloma virus (HPV), chlamydia, and gonorrhea. Some STDs are caused by bacteria (B), or viruses (V), or parasites (P). Research online about each STD's method of transmission and symptoms.

	STDs	Transmission	Symptoms
1)	human papilloma virus (V)		
2)	chlamydia (B)		
3)	gonorrhea (B)		
4)	genital herpes (V)		
5)	hepatitis B (V)		
6)	syphilis (B)		
7)	HIV (V)		
8)	pubic lice (P)		
9)	trichomoniasis (P)		
10)	mononucleosis (V)		

E Pair and Share #2

Compare your answers from Section D with a classmate. Which answers are the same? Which answers are different? Discuss and decide which one you are most surprised about. Give reasons to support your thinking.

A: I didn't know gonorrhea was caused by bacteria.

B: Yeah, and I also thought you could catch it by kissing. I was wrong.

EXTENSIONS ➡ How does sexual health education in Japan compare with other countries?

_____

_____

022
2-8

In 1981, clinicians in the US grew concerned when previously healthy **homosexual** (gay) men began presenting with **pneumocystis pneumonia** (PCP), a rare and **opportunistic infection (OI)**. While this was not the origin of AIDS, it was the beginning of what would become the AIDS epidemic in the US. The origin was said to be in Central Africa as early as
5 the late 1800s. Human immunodeficiency virus (HIV), a **retrovirus** that causes AIDS, is a zoonotic virus which was first passed to humans from chimpanzees infected with the **simian immunodeficiency virus (SIV)**. It was thought to be transferred to humans by contact with infected meat and blood products.

HIV was first reported in Japan in 1984 and considered a foreign disease brought back
10 by travelers from overseas. However, investigations revealed that **hemophiliacs** were infected with contaminated blood as early as 1982. Though HIV was initially considered a "gay disease," increasing PCP and OI infections in **heterosexuals**, hemophiliacs, and even infants emphasized to the medical community that HIV can affect anyone. It was not long before HIV was declared a sexually transmitted disease (STD).

15 HIV is generally spread through sexual intercourse or sharing needles. There are two major indicators for HIV, one is **T-cell count** and the other is **viral load**. The HIV virus impacts T-cell count, particularly T-cells that carry the CD4 protein on their surface. There are many types of CD4 T-cells, including helper, regulatory and memory T-cells; these are major components of both the innate and adaptive immune systems. HIV progressively
20 destroys these CD4 T-cells. The **CD4 count** is used to indicate the stages of HIV infection. A normal CD4 count ranges from 500-1500 cells/mm^3 of blood. If it drops below 200 cells, it is a sign of AIDS (3rd stage) and drastically increases the body's susceptibility to OIs. Viral load is the measure of how much virus is in the blood and is indicative of transmissibility. The aim of treatment is to reduce the viral load to less than 50 copies/ml. In the genetic material
25 of most animals, DNA is used to create RNA, which is then read to create proteins. HIV, however, is a retrovirus. Retro, meaning backwards, refers to reverse transcription; HIV starts with RNA, using this to create DNA. **Antiretroviral therapy**, known as **ART**, is used to effectively treat HIV infections.

Fast-forward 40 years and the development of new and better treatments for HIV has
30 come a long way. Though 38 million people are currently living with HIV worldwide, in the developed world, life expectancy for someone with HIV is now similar to someone who is not infected with the virus. This continues to depend on timing of diagnosis, access to good health care, and adherence to medication regimens; in cases with late diagnosis, the prognosis is less promising. These days if someone unknowingly has HIV and donates blood, strict
35 screening programs are in place to identify the infection and remove it from the blood supply.

In 2020, HIV/AIDS cases in Japan had decreased from previous years to 1085 persons, 55 of whom were women. There are concerns that the number of new cases may actually be higher due to a lack of testing during the COVID-19 pandemic, but time will tell. There is still a need to update education programs with the latest information in schools and **disseminate**

40 information in the community so that people are well informed and to prevent discrimination and forced disclosures.

🔊 Words and Phrases

homosexual 同性愛の
pneumocystis pneumonia ニューモシスチス肺炎
opportunistic infection (OI) 日和見感染症
retrovirus レトロウイルス
simian immunodeficiency virus (SIV) 類人猿免疫不全ウイルス
hemophiliacs 血友病患者
heterosexuals 異性愛者

T-cell count T 細胞数
viral load ウイルス量、ウイルス負荷
CD4 count CD4 数
antiretroviral therapy (ART)
　抗レトロウイルス療法
disseminate （情報・知識・考えなどを）広める、
　普及させる

Language Advice   Greek and Latin

Knowing the origin of words and the meaning of their parts can help you understand them. Some examples include:

infectious   Latin – *inficere/infection/infectus* – to put in, stain, dye
zoonotic   Greek – *zoon* – animal, *nosos* – disease
epidemic   Greek – *epi* - on, *demos* – people
pandemic   Greek – *pan* – all, *demos* – people

Ⓖ Research #2 – Anatomy

a) Work alone. What parts of the body are affected in the 3 stages of HIV/AIDs? Write your answers on the right-hand side. If you do NOT know an answer, leave it blank. NOTE In part (a) do NOT look online for the answers.

b) After, work with a partner and discuss your answers. Fill in any of the answers you are missing.

c) Next, work with your partner and check your answers online.

d) Finally, your teacher will give you the answers. Check to see if your answers are correct.

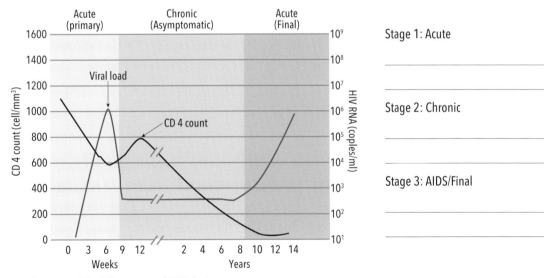

An illustration of the diffrent stages of HIV infection.

Source: Manoto, Sello & Lugongolo, Masixole & Govender, Ureshnie & Mthunzi-Kufa, Patience. (2018). Point of Care Diagnostics for HIV in Resource Limited Settings: An Overview. Medicina. 54. 3. 10.3390/medicina54010003.

H Research #3 – Group Work

Make a team of 3-4 members. HIV/AIDs treatment, ART, affects people differently and there are several known side effects. Research online about these side effects. After each team is finished, share your answers.

Side effects:

_____

_____

EXTENSIONS ➡ Penicillin is a well-known antibiotic. Why was it called "the wonder drug"?

_____

_____

I Discussion – Should Workers Have to Declare Their HIV Status?

A 2020 newspaper article in Japan reported that an employee was forced to disclose his HIV status. At his workplace, the employee's superior introduced him to the other workers as being infected with HIV. However, government guidelines state that workers should not be disadvantaged because of their HIV status. What is your opinion?

a) Work with a team of 3-4 members. Discuss if workers should have to declare their HIV status.
b) After discussing in your team, vote on whether you agree or disagree? Be prepared to give reasons for your viewpoint.

Agree	Disagree

J Project – STDs

a) Work with a group of 3-4 members. Choose one of the STDs from the list below and research about it:

☐ human papilloma virus (HPV)   ☐ trichomoniasis   ☐ HTLV
☐ gonorrhea   ☐ chlamydia   ☐ mononucleosis
☐ hepatitis B   ☐ genital herpes
☐ HIV   ☐ syphilis

b) Create a team PPT to share what you have learned. Include the following information in your PPT:

- What is the definition of the STD?
- Is the chosen STD viral or bacterial?
- How is it diagnosed?
- What are the symptoms and treatment?
- What is the prognosis?
- Who is the target group(s)?
- Include photos, illustrations, and/or diagrams to support your research.
- Include references, showing where you found the information online.

 Presentation Skills – How to Improve Your Eye Contact

Although it is very stressful for some presenters, making appropriate eye contact with your audience is important during a presentation. Below is some advice to help improve your eye contact:

1) Finish preparing your presentation a few days BEFORE the date you will present.
2) Practice! This means standing up, speaking out loud, and make eye contact with the imaginary audience (or even yourself in front of a mirror). Imagine you are in front of a group of people who are listening to your talk. The more you know your presentation, the more you can improve your eye contact.
3) During an audience presentation: Look at the listeners in the room in a "Z" pattern, moving across the front row, through the middle, and across the back.
4) During a poster presentation: Look at each person who is listening to your talk long enough to make a comfortable connection (3-5 seconds).
5) During an online presentation: Look at the camera on your computer (not yourself on video).
6) Remember, you don't need to look at the audience 100% of the time. It is ok to look away and point to interesting information on your PPT (PowerPoint) or your poster as you speak.

EXTENSIONS

a) Work with the same team members from Section J.
b) Do "Rock, Paper, Scissors."
c) The winner: Read the passage below.
d) The listeners: Score the reader's eye contact using the scoring scale below.
e) Repeat until each member has had a turn.

Fast-forward 40 years and the development of new and better treatments for HIV has come a long way. Though 38 million people are currently living with HIV worldwide, in the developed world, life expectancy for someone with HIV is now similar to someone who is not infected with the virus.

Eye Contact Scoring Scale
Great = Nearly always making eye contact   Good = ~ 50% of the time
Poor =   Little or no eye contact

L **Reflection**

Work alone. Think back over what you have learned in this unit and record your answers below.

1) What are some interesting things you have learned in this unit?
2) What do you want to improve about your learning?
3) If you did a presentation, what went well? What did not?

Allergies

A What Do You Know?

What do you know about allergies? Write 3 ideas below.

1) _____

_____

2) _____

_____

3) _____

_____

B Pair and Share #1

Talk with a partner and share your ideas from Section A. Remember to ask follow-up questions or make comments as your partner shares their answers:

- Wow!
- Why do you think that?
- That's a good point.
- Hmmm…that sounds logical.

C Paired Listening

a) Work with a partner. Listen to a teacher's talk about allergies. Take notes as you listen and answer the questions below.

1) What is one allergen that is found in the home?
2) What is the allergen found in pets called?
3) What illness has cockroach allergens been linked to?
4) What are 2 things you can do to reduce mold in your home?

b) Work with a partner and check your answers.

EXTENSIONS ▶ Based on the listening, what allergens do you think can be found in your house or apartment? What can be done to reduce or eliminate them?

_____

_____

D Research #1 – Common Allergies

Allergies are one of the most common forms of chronic disease. In addition to this, the number of allergy sufferers are increasing worldwide year by year. What are some of the most common allergens worldwide? What are some of the most common in Japan? Research online and make a list below.

What are some of the most common allergens worldwide?	What are some of the most common allergens in Japan?
1)	1)
2)	2)
3)	3)
4)	4)
5)	5)
6)	6)
7)	7)
8)	8)
9)	9)
10)	10)

E Pair and Share #2

Compare your answers from Section D with a classmate. Which answers are the same? Which answers are different? Which allergen do you think is the most common worldwide? How about in Japan? Give reasons to support your thinking.

A: Which allergen do you think is the most common worldwide?
B: I thought peanuts were the most common allergen. How about you?

EXTENSIONS ➡ What is the most common allergy in Japan? Is it unique to Japan?

F Reading – Allergies

Worldwide, allergies are one of the most common chronic diseases, and the number of people who have allergies is increasing each year. The severity of allergies can range from mild symptoms to life threatening reactions. What exactly are allergies and who can be affected by them? What are the symptoms? Are there any treatments available?

5   The body's immune system works to combat invaders outside the body, like viruses and

bacteria. However, your body may have an exaggerated reaction to a harmless substance (called an allergen), which may not cause a reaction in another person. Examples of allergens include nuts, pollen, animal **dander**, and bee venom after a sting. Potential allergens can also be found in some places you might not think of, such as the nickel in clothing fasteners and jewelry, and the latex found in some gloves and other products.

People react to allergens in different ways, but why only certain people have allergies is not completely known. We do know that allergies are more common in children than adults, but allergies can develop at any point in a person's life. Also, sometimes the allergies we have in childhood disappear later in life. If you have a parent who has had allergies, your chances to have allergies are increased, but not all allergies are **hereditary** (like allergies to **penicillin** or shellfish). Your chances of having an allergy may also be linked to your environment. For example, some evidence suggests that being around pets as a young child may help make your body more **resilient** to allergens as an adult. Other data suggests that children who grow up being exposed to a greater variety of microbes in their natural environment may have more flexible immune systems when faced with allergic triggers compared to children who live in urban settings and who are not as exposed to these microbes.

Some people suffer from the seasonal allergy commonly known as hay fever (also known as allergic rhinitis or AR). The symptoms can be mild but may affect the whole body. Common symptoms of hay fever include a runny nose, itchy eyes and throat, and sinus congestion. More **systemic** symptoms may include headaches or fatigue and rashes. However, sometimes an allergic reaction can be much more severe and cause life-threatening symptoms. Medicines like penicillin, venom from bee or wasp stings, and some kinds of food can trigger a severe reaction in some people. These reactions can include hives, swelling, difficulty in breathing, and a fall in blood pressure, which together are known as **anaphylaxis**. Anaphylaxis can happen seconds or minutes after exposure to an allergen, forcing your body into anaphylactic shock. Without medical treatment, such as an epinephrine injection, anaphylaxis can be fatal for some people.

Although allergies cannot be totally cured yet, there are steps you can take to ease the symptoms. For example, in the case of hay fever, as well as dust **mite** and animal dander allergies, keeping your home clean and free of carpets, down quilts, and feather pillows, all of which can collect allergens, is recommended. During seasons with high pollen counts (pollen season), limiting your exposure to the outdoors, wearing a mask and eye protection, and closing your windows are other preventive measures. In addition to these behavioral measures, there are various **over-the-counter (OTC) drugs**, such as **antihistamines** and **decongestants**, that can help reduce your symptoms, as well as several prescription medications. Some natural remedies are also available. For example, for hay fever, natural treatments may include honey, garlic, hot peppers, chamomile tea, and taking a shower.

It should be mentioned that in Japan, hay fever from cedar pollen is listed as one of the most common allergies. This is probably due to widespread planting of cedar trees after World War II. The number of people in Japan suffering from hay fever continues to rise each year.

◇ Words and Phrases

dander 鱗屑（動物の毛や羽からはがれ落ちたもの）	anaphylaxis アナフィラキシー、過敏反応
hereditary 遺伝	mite ダニ
penicillin ペニシリン	over-the-counter (OTC) （医者の処方箋なしで）薬が店頭売買される
resilient 回復の早い	antihistamines 抗ヒスタミン剤
systemic 全身性の	decongestants （鼻炎などの）充血緩和剤、消炎剤

Language Point   **Borrowed Words**

Japanese, like other languages, has borrowed words. Below are a few medical words that come from the German language.

Japanese	German	English		Japanese	German	English
アレルギー	Allergie	allergy		ジフィリス	Syphilis	syphilis
ウイルス／ビールス	Virus	virus		カルテ	Karte	chart; medical record
エネルギー	Energie	energy		レントゲン	Röntgen	X-ray
ギプス	Gips	plaster cast; cast		ワクチン	Vakzin	vaccine (shot, jab)

G   **Research #2 – Anatomy**

a) Work alone. Think about anaphylaxis. Fill in the missing symptoms that match each system. If you do NOT know an answer, leave it blank. NOTE In part (a) do NOT look online for the answers.

b) After, work with a partner and discuss your answers. Fill in any of the answers you are missing.

c) Next, work with your partner and check your answers online.

d) Finally, your teacher will give you the answers. Check to see if your answers are correct.

Anaphylaxis	Systems	Symptoms
	1 Skin	1) _____
	2 Respiratory	2) _____
	3 Gastrointestinal	3) _____
	4 Cardiovascular	4) _____
	5 Neurological	5) _____

based on https://www.medicalestudy.com/acute-anaphylaxis-signssymptoms-treatment/

H Research #3 – Group Work

Make a team of 3-4 members. Besides <u>pollen</u> which causes <u>hay fever</u>, choose an allergy trigger and research about it online. Be sure to answer each of the questions below as you research. After each team is finished, share your answers.

Allergy Trigger: _____

- What are the symptoms?
- What are the risk factors?
- What are some complications?
- What are some treatments or prevention?

EXTENSIONS Seasonal allergies and having a cold have some of the same symptoms. Which symptoms are the same? Which are different?

_____

_____

I Discussion – How Can Seasonal Pollen Allergies Be Managed?

During the Meiji period through World War II, Japan's forests were depleted for lumber used for building. After World War II, 40% of Japanese forests were replanted with cedar and cypress trees. Although these trees grew quickly and reforested empty forestlands, they also became mass producers of pollen when they reached maturity 30 years later. Since the 1960s, the number of people who suffer from hay fever has increased year by year. What can be done to manage seasonal pollen allergies in Japan? What can people do at home? What can science do to help reduce seasonal pollen?

Work with a team of 3-4 members. Research and discuss a plan to manage or reduce hay fever. Take notes about your plan in the box below. After hearing each team's presentation, which team(s) has the best approach?

NOTES

Project – PPT Infographic

Work with a group of 3-4 members. As a team, research and create a 5-slide PPT infographic about hay fever, covering the following points:

- What are the symptoms?
- What are the risk factors?
- What are some complications?
- What are some treatments or prevention?
- What natural remedies can be used?

 Presentation Skills – Gestures

What should you do with your hands during a presentation? This is a common worry for some presenters. Instead of standing and holding your notes, try using some gestures in your next presentation. Gestures can make your talk more attractive for the listener and make your information more understandable. Below is some advice to help you add gestures to your presentation:

1) Adding some gestures is a great idea, but too many and you will look unnatural.
2) Add gestures to emphasize your talking points.
3) Practice your presentation to understand where your gestures will work the best.
4) Film yourself or practice in front of a friend to get feedback.
5) Look online and watch other presenters to find some of the best kinds of gestures for your presentation.
6) Although there are many different gestures, some useful ones include:
   - Pointing to your information (but do not point at your audience)
   - Listing/counting on your fingers
   - Showing size or comparisons (this or that; big or small; increase or decrease)
   - Gesturing with your palms up (this can help show that the speaker is non-threatening)

EXTENSIONS →

a) Work with the same team members from Section J.
b) Project your team's PPT on a screen.
c) Select one member to share 2 points from the PPT.
d) Presenter: Share 2 points from your PPT with gestures. Think to yourself which gestures can you include to make your talk more interesting?
e) Listeners: Give praise and feedback.
f) Switch roles and have another presenter share 2 points with gestures. Repeat until each member has had a turn.

 Reflection

Work alone. Think back over what you have learned in this unit and record your answers below.

1) What are some interesting things you have learned in this unit?
2) What do you want to improve about your learning?
3) If you did a presentation, what went well? What did not?

Environmental Health Issues

A What Do You Know?

What do you know about environmental health issues? Write 3 ideas below.

1) _____

_____

2) _____

_____

3) _____

_____

B Pair and Share #1

Talk with a partner and share your ideas from Section A. Remember to ask follow-up questions or make comments as your partner shares their answers:

- That's interesting! What else do you know about…?
- Wow! Where did you hear that?
- That makes sense to me.
- Here are my three ideas.

C Paired Listening

025
2-11

a) Work with a partner. Listen to a classroom teacher talk about environmental health issues. Take notes as you listen and answer the questions below.

1) What four environmental health factors are mentioned by the teacher?
2) Which environmental diseases are associated with the highest mortality amongst children worldwide?

b) Work with a partner and check your answers.

EXTENSIONS ➡ Do you think it is safe to drink tap water in Japan? Why or why not? Can you think of any situations in which it would become unsafe to drink tap water in Japan?

_____

_____

D   Research #1 – Environmental Factors

Our surroundings are often an indicator of our overall health and well-being. Research online and make a list of 10 environmental factors that can cause disease. Do NOT forget to list the diseases and health risks that can be caused by each factor.

Environmental Factors	Diseases/Health Risks
1)	
2)	
3)	
4)	
5)	
6)	
7)	
8)	
9)	
10)	

E   Pair and Share #2

Compare your answers from Section D with a classmate. Which answers are the same? Which answers are different? Discuss and decide which environmental factor has the biggest impact on global health. Give reasons to support your thinking.

A: I think air pollution is the most dangerous to global health, as it is thought to cause the most deaths worldwide. Every year, millions of deaths are linked to air pollution, mainly from heart disease, stroke, and chronic obstructive pulmonary disease (COPD).

B: I have a different opinion. I chose water pollution because of the devastating impact it has on children's health. Contaminated water causes diarrhea and parasitic diseases in children, contributing to chronic malnutrition and starvation.

EXTENSIONS ➡ What do you think is the most serious environmental issue in Japan? Why?

Climate change refers to long-term shifts in temperatures and weather patterns. These shifts can occur naturally, but for the past two centuries human activities appear to be the main driver of climate change. Activities like burning fossil fuels (such as coal, oil, and gas), deforestation, and increased livestock farming have all contributed to producing heat-trapping

5 gases (called the greenhouse effect). It is worth noting that according to the World Health Organization (WHO), climate change is the single biggest health threat that humanity faces.

Although some of the more obvious health effects of climate change include individual injuries, illnesses, and premature deaths due to extreme weather, climate change has also had an adverse effect on communities and our environment worldwide. Climate change has

10 altered patterns of infectious and parasitic disease, often by extending their boundaries. It has also damaged **agricultural production**, contributing to an estimated 150,000 deaths annually due to malnutrition. Increases in climate change-related air pollution and **vector-borne diseases** have had an even more devastating impact on global health. Urban air pollution generated by vehicles, industry, and energy production kills approximately 800,000

15 people annually, while malaria kills over 1.2 million, mostly children in Africa under the age of five.

Statistics indicate that the health burden caused by climate change will mainly fall on developing countries, particularly on poor children who are more vulnerable to climate-related diseases such as asthma and infectious diseases like malaria and water-borne illnesses.

20 However, the effects of climate change can be felt in **affluent** countries too, from heatwaves and increased rainfall in Japan to droughts and forest fires in California and Australia. Regardless of region or status, climate change is perhaps the biggest health challenge that humankind faces.

What needs to be done? For the long-term health of humanity, transformational action

25 must be taken to reduce emissions and avoid breaking through dangerous temperature **thresholds**. According to a special report by the United Nations (UN), by 2030, global carbon dioxide emissions must be 45% less than they were in 2010, and reach net zero by 2075. One way this can be achieved is by planting more trees and utilizing **carbon capture and storage** technologies. In addition, shifting to renewable energies, changing in our habits

30 of food consumption to decrease land-intensive animal products, and electrifying transport are some of the best investments to protect generational global health.

◦ Words and Phrases

agricultural production 農業生産物	threshold 境界、閾の
vector-borne diseases ベクター媒介性疾患	carbon capture and storage 二酸化炭素の回収と貯蓄
affluent 裕福な	

In English there are many different rules for plural nouns, usually depending on what letter a word ends in. Irregular nouns do not follow plural noun rules, so they must be memorized. Here are some of the most common patterns:

Regular nouns: add-S   physicians, patients, hospitals, vaccines
Ends in consonant + Y: remove Y, add -IES   surgeries, injuries, therapies
Ends in S, CH, SH, X or Z: add -ES   stresses, crutches, appendixes

G Research #2 – Anatomy

a) Work alone. Look at the list of body systems. Write down the illnesses/injures associated with toxic chemical exposure for each of the body systems. If you do NOT know an answer, leave it blank.
NOTE In part (a) do NOT look online for the answers.
b) After, work with a partner and discuss your answers. Fill in any of the answers you are missing.
c) Next, work with your partner and check your answers online.
d) Finally, your teacher will give you the answers. Check to see if your answers are correct.

Body Systems	Illnesses/Injuries Associated with Toxic Chemical Exposure
The cardiovascular system	
The nervous system	
The immune system	
The reproductive system	
The respiratory system	
The integumentary (skin) system	

H Research #3 – Group Work

Make a team of 3-4 members. Choose one body system from Section G and research its functions. Then, research ways this body system is affected by climate change. After each team is finished, share your answers.

System: _____
Functions:
_____
_____

Ways the body system is affected by climate change:
_____
_____

EXTENSIONS ➡ What is the most common illness or injury associated with toxic chemical exposure? Research online and find the answers.

_____

_____

Ⅰ Discussion – Are Food Additives Safe?

Food additives are chemicals that keep foods fresh or enhance their color, flavor, or texture. Some of the most common food additives are monosodium glutamate (MSG), high-fructose corn syrup, and artificial food dyes. Food additives are also the subject of intense debate: Are food additives dangerous toxins or marvels of science?

Work with a team of 3-4 members. Discuss the safety of food additives. Do they positively or negatively affect our health? After discussing, decide with your team if you support the use of food additives or not.

Good Points	Bad Points

Ⅰ Project – A Study of Environmental Health Issues by Country

a) Work with a group of 3-4 members. Choose one of the countries from the list below.

☐ Bangladesh   ☐ Canada   ☐ Germany   ☐ Haiti   ☐ Japan
☐ Mongolia   ☐ Nigeria   ☐ Qatar   ☐ Rwanda

84

b) Create a PPT and include the following information in your presentation:

- Introduce the country (name, location, language, capital, population, weather, gross domestic product (GDP)).
- What is the state of water quality?
- What is the air quality index (AQI) of this country?
- Which infectious diseases are a problem in this country (e.g., malaria, tuberculosis, HIV/AIDS, COVID-19)?
- Is infrastructure (roads, railroads, ports, airports) a problem in this country? In what way(s)?
- How has climate change affected this country?

K Presentation Skills – Q&A

For some presenters, it can be very stressful answering questions after your presentation. To avoid feeling too much anxiety, here are some tips to help improve your Q&A session as part of your next presentation:
1) Anticipate the most likely questions you might receive at the end of your talk. Think about what information that you need to share to clarify any points that might be unclear to the audience.
2) Thank the audience member for asking a question.
3) Listen to the question; do not be afraid to rephrase it or repeat it back, especially if you need to clarify the meaning, or because you could not hear the audience member.
4) Hold back some information; you do not need to include everything in your presentation, especially if it will become overly complicated. Additional points can be shared in more detail in the Q&A session.
5) Decide when you will take questions. Some people take questions during their presentations, others at the end, and some (especially for long and details answers) take them in the lobby after the talk.

EXTENSIONS
a) Work with the same team members from Section J.
b) Do "Rock, Paper, Scissors."
c) The winner: Briefly share one of the subtopics from your PPT in Section J.
d) The listeners: Each member asks one question.
e) The winner: Follow the tips above and answer the questions.
f) Repeat until each member has had a turn.

L Reflection

Work alone. Think back over what you have learned in this unit and record your answers below.

1) What are some interesting things you have learned in this unit?
2) What do you want to improve about your learning?
3) If you did a presentation, what went well? What did not?

CAM (Complementary and Alternative Medicine)

A What Do You Know?

What do you know about CAM (Complementary and Alternative Medicine)? Write 3 ideas below.

1) _____

_____

2) _____

_____

3) _____

_____

B Pair and Share #1

Talk with a partner and share your ideas from Section A. Remember to ask follow-up questions or make comments as your partner shares their answers:

- Do you know anything about...?
- I think that _____ might be like...
- Oh really? Is it like/Is it similar to...?
- When did you hear that?

C Paired Listening

027
2-13

a) Work with a partner. Listen to a health professional describing one kind of CAM. Take notes as you listen and answer the questions below.

1) What kind of CAM is the person talking about?
2) What condition was it used for?
3) How many treatments did they have?
4) What are the lines along the body called?

b) Work with a partner and check your answers.

EXTENSIONS ➡ How many bones are there in the shoulder joint? What are the rotator cuff muscles? What range of movement is normal for the shoulder?

_____

_____

What are 10 kinds of CAM therapies? Research online and make a list below. Categorize each into the appropriate column based on whether it is a physical/tactile therapy or medicinal/oral therapy. The first one has been done for you.

CAM	Physical/Tactile Therapy	Medicinal/Oral Therapy
acupuncture	✓	

E Pair and Share #2

Compare your answers from Section D with a classmate. Which answers are the same? Which answers are different? Discuss and decide which one you are most interested in from each of your lists. Give reasons to support your thinking.

A: Are you more interested in tactile therapies or oral CAM therapies?

B: I'm more interested in tactile ones, particularly aromatherapy massage. My friend tried it and said it was really relaxing. How about you?

EXTENSIONS ➡ Which body or organ systems are affected by CAM? How many different systems are there?

_____

_____

How did people heal or cure themselves before the advent of modern medicine? Looking back through history, it is easy to identify "folk medicine" traditions in most cultures, which describe how a variety of plants and other natural substances were used for reducing a fever or dressing a wound. Some of these traditions were oral, such as indigenous Australian "bush
5   medicine", which was passed down by word of mouth from generation to generation, while others were written down, such as India's Ayurvedic texts that date back more than 5,000 years.

In recent times, with the advent of modern technology, the average person can find an enormous amount of information on the internet. This is also true of healthcare information.
10   Nowadays, virtually anyone can research the best treatment for a particular health condition, find a highly-skilled specialist, or a hospital that has the latest **cutting-edge technology**. Nonetheless, according to the United States' Institute of Medicine, the number of people who are becoming interested in natural therapies is on the rise. These therapies are sometimes referred to as **CAM**. However, what exactly is CAM?

15   CAM stands for Complementary and Alternative Medicine. Therapies which fall under this **umbrella term**, for example acupuncture and osteopathy, have been considered at one time or another outside of the conventional Western medical model of treatment. In other words, they have historically not been accepted or studied alongside **allopathy**. Even today, many of these treatments are labeled "alternative", and in some cases have even been
20   considered dangerous compared to conventional medicine.

However, as many of these therapies have become more well-known, some even having received formal certification for their practice and gained insurance coverage (in some countries), they are being increasingly sought after by patients. An increasing number of physicians are even using these modalities in conjunction with allopathic medicine. In the
25   latter situation, these therapies are often referred to as complimentary, meaning they can be incorporated or used together with conventional therapies. A survey of Japanese doctors in 2011 discovered that 52% regularly prescribed *kampo* (traditional Chinese herbal medicine) to their patients.

There is a general feeling that CAM offers a holistic approach compared to regular
30   medicine, but definitions vary as to what therapies can be included under this term. A general method for categorizing CAM therapies has been established in the US. In 2000, the National Centre for Complementary and Alternative Medicine (NCCAM) suggested 5 categories to help classify the large number of CAM. The five categories are **manipulative** and body-based methods; mind-body **interventions**; alternative medical systems; energy therapies;
35   and biologically-based treatments.

These days, at the educational level, it is now possible to study acupuncture, Chinese

medicine, chiropractic and osteopathy at the same university (such as RMIT in Melbourne, Australia). Previously, it was not uncommon for medical professionals to have to travel to China to study acupuncture! Along with allopathic medical schools, many training institutions
40 now also offer clinical sites where trainees can practice CAM skills. This suggests that the world of mainstream medicine and complementary medicine are coexisting with some degree of recognition and acceptance. Therefore, it is beneficial for healthcare providers to be familiar with the broad range of CAM. When patients confide that they are using some form of CAM, an astute provider can offer support, such as confirming whether or not it is in the
45 patient's best interest to continue the therapy.

Words and Phrases

cutting-edge technology 先端技術
CAM (Complementary and Alternative Medicine) 補完代替医療
umbrella term 包括的用語

allopathy 逆症療法
manipulative 整復の
intervention 介入

Language Advice **Word Pair Opposites**

Word pair opposites are useful when describing pros and cons in medical situations.

- beneficial - detrimental
- benefits - drawbacks
- upside - downside
- advantages - disadvantages
- alleviate - aggravate

G **Research #2 – Common CAM Categories**

a) Work alone. Identify the CAM therapies that fall into each of the 5 CAM categories. If you do NOT know an answer, leave it blank. NOTE In part (a) do NOT look online for the answers.
b) After, work with a partner and discuss your answers. Fill in any of the answers you are missing.
c) Next, work with your partner and check your answers online.
d) Finally, your teacher will give you the answers. Check to see if your answers are correct.

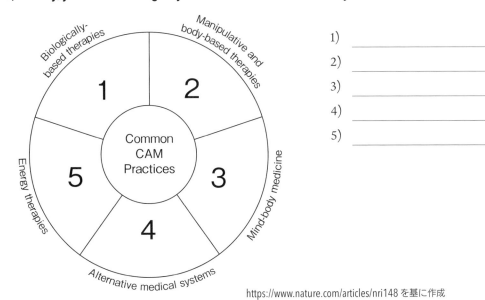

1) _____
2) _____
3) _____
4) _____
5) _____

https://www.nature.com/articles/nri148 を基に作成

H Research #3 – Group Work

Make a team of 3-4 members. Choose one of the CAM therapies from Section G and research about its effects on a particular illness/disease. After each team is finished, share your answers.

CAM Treatment	Illness	Result

EXTENSIONS ➡ Consider the results from a physiological perspective. What is happening at the cellular level? Can you explain it? Research online and find the answers.

I Discussion – Opinions About CAM

a) Work with a team of 3-4 members. What do you think of the statement below? Discuss what the statement means.

> "National Institutes of Health (NIH) studies have shown that acupuncture is an effective treatment alone or in combination with conventional therapies."
>
> https://www.hopkinsmedicine.org/health/wellness-and-prevention/acupuncture

b) Afterward, research other CAM online. What are some opinions about its use in health care? Discuss your findings with your team. Be prepared to give reasons for your viewpoint.

CAM	Opinions About CAM	Your viewpoint

J Project – Advice for Patients Using CAM in Conjunction with Conventional Medicine

a) Work with a group of 3-4 members. Fill in the table below.

b) One of your patients is curious about CAM.

c) First, offer some general advice to your patient about using CAM.

d) Next, List three kinds of therapies and specific advice about those therapies.

e) After, research online and check if your ideas are correct.

General CAM Advice	CAM	CAM	CAM
	Specific Advice	Specific Advice	Specific Advice

e) Create a team PPT about CAM to share what you have learned. Include the following information in your PPT:

- Choose one CAM
- The body system(s) involved
- How it works
- Any data to support its effectiveness
- Generalized advice
- Specific advice regarding the chosen CAM
- Include photos, illustrations and/or diagrams to support your research
- Include references showing where you found the information online

In the era of virtual meetings, it is more than likely you will give a presentation via a virtual platform (such as Zoom, Webex, or Google Meet) in the future. Below is some advice to help improve your virtual presentations online:

1) Use Visual Aids

Audiences love visual aids; they make it easier for listeners to quickly process your main message and remember content. For a visually appealing and engaging presentation, include images and videos to explain how things work and emphasize your important ideas. Use visual data in the form of charts and graphs to effectively display numbers.

2) Be Seen and Heard

What an audience can see and hear hugely impacts the effectiveness of a presentation. To appear as professional as possible, good lighting conditions are vital. Natural light is the best tool to look good during a virtual presentation. Make sure you sit near a window, but avoid having it behind your back as it will create a shadow. To provide a better visual experience for the audience, frame yourself correctly. Make sure your camera is at eye level with the presenter, and not tilted forward or backward. Your head should be in the top 50% of the frame so the audience can see your shoulders and any hand gestures you make during the presentation.

To improve your audio quality, use earbuds or a headset; computer microphones may be too far away to pick up your voice clearly. Close windows and doors to keep your location as quiet and free of ambient noise as possible. A final quick audio tip is to avoid overloading your device; close any unnecessary applications and browser tabs during your presentation.

3) Engage with Your Audience

One of the top tips is to stick something eye-catching next to your device's camera to help maintain eye contact with the audience. Also, keep your audience engaged by utilizing the interactive functions on your platform's software. Integrate the chat function or launch a poll to help boost audience participation. Breakout rooms are an excellent choice for online workshops or training sessions. Participants can discuss the topics from your presentation in greater detail and express their ideas, allowing for a more collaborative and memorable experience.

EXTENSIONS ➡

a) Work with the same team members from Section J.
b) Open the link to watch a short Zoom presentation: https://www.youtube.com/watch?v=Uo0Wg3OD4Nc Watch the presentation as a group.
c) Did the presentation follow the tips for virtual presenting? What were its strengths and weaknesses? Discuss with your group.

 Reflection

Work alone. Think back over what you have learned in this unit and record your answers below.

1) What are some interesting things you have learned in this unit?
2) What do you want to improve about your learning?
3) If you did a presentation, what went well? What did not?

Glossary

A
acute
adaptive immunity
affluent
agricultural production
allopathy
anaphylaxis
antihistamines
antiretroviral therapy (ART)
autonomy

B
behavior therapy
binge
biopsy
bone marrow
brain shrinkage

C
CAM (Complementary and Alternative Medicine)
carbohydrates (carbs)
carbon capture and storage
CD4 count
cholesterol
chronic
chronic constipation
circadian rhythms
circulation
cognition
cognitive functioning
cognitive process
compulsive
cutting-edge technology

D
dander
decongestants
dendritic cells
dependency
deteriorate
differentiate
disseminate
dopamine

E
EEG

efficacy
empty calories raise the risk for/lead to
epidemic
executive function

F
fatigue
femur
forced disclosures
fuse

G
gastroesophageal reflux disease (GERD)
genes

H
HDL
hemophiliacs
hereditary
heterosexuals
homosexual
hygiene

I
incentive salience
incus
inhibit
inhibitions
innate immunity
intervention
irritable bowel syndrome (IBS)

J
jellyfish

K
kidneys

L
LDL
lethargy
leukocytes
lipoprotein
liver
low-impact aerobic exercise

M

malleus
manipulative
menopausal
meta-studies
metabolic syndrome
mites
mobility
morbidity
mortality
mortality rate
mutation

N

neural
neurology
neurotransmitter
non-communicable
NREM

O

obese
obesity
obstetrician
opportunistic infection (OI)
osteoporosis
over-the-counter (OTC)
oxalates

P

pancreas
paralysis
participant
penicillin
perfectionism
persistent
pessimistic
phytates
pineal gland
pneumocystis pneumonia
polio
pollutants
porous
prevalence
protein biomarkers
psychotherapy
puberty

Q

quality of life (QOL)

R

randomized control trials (RCTs)
REM
resilient
retrovirus
rubella

S

sedentary
simian immunodeficiency virus (SIV)
social engagement
socioeconomic status
stage
stapes
stave off
stooped
stressors
substance
systemic

T

T-cell count
threshold
triglycerides

U

umbrella term

V

vector-borne diseases
viral load
vivid
vulnerable

W

workaholic

Z

zoonotic

REFERENCES

[Unit 1]

F.

https://www.otsuka.co.jp/en/nutraceutical/about/nutrition/functions/

https://www.helpguide.org/articles/healthy-eating/choosing-healthy-carbs.htm

https://www.medicalnewstoday.com/articles/219305

https://www.niddk.nih.gov/health-information/digestive-diseases/digestive-system-how-it-works

https://www.nippon.com/en/japan-data/h00853/

K.

https://www.mayoclinic.org/diseases-conditions/specific-phobias/expert-answers/fear-of-public-speaking/faq-20058416

https://www.mentalhelp.net/blogs/what-we-fear-more-than-death/

https://www.genardmethod.com/blog/10-fast-and-effective-ways-to-overcome-stage-fright

https://corporatecommunicationexperts.com.au/6-tips-deal-stage-fright/

[Unit 2]

https://www.mayoclinic.org/healthy-lifestyle/fitness/in-depth/fitness/art-20045099

https://www.mayoclinic.org/healthy-lifestyle/fitness/in-depth/aerobic-exercise/art-20045541

https://www.healthline.com/health/high-cholesterol/foods-to-increase-hdl

https://www.nhs.uk/live-well/exercise/exercise-health-benefits/

https://www.nhs.uk/conditions/sports-injuries/

https://en.wikipedia.org/wiki/Physical_fitness

[Unit 3]

E.

Extension: https://www.sciencedaily.com/releases/2014/12/141222165033.htm

F.

Facts & wording

https://www.bidmc.org/about-bidmc/wellness-insights/bones-and-joints/2018/08/fun-facts-about-bones-and-joints

http://www.bonehealthandosteoporosis.org/wp-content/uploads/2016/04/Healthy-Bone-Brochure_FINAL.pdf

https://www.mayoclinic.org/healthy-lifestyle/adult-health/in-depth/bone-health/art-20045060

https://www.mayoclinic.org/diseases-conditions/osteoporosis/symptoms-causes/syc-20351968

https://www.sportsmed.org/aossmimis/STOP/Downloads/SportsTips/ExerciseBoneHealth.pdf

https://www.osteoporosis.foundation/patients/about-osteoporosis?utm_source=Enigma&utm_medium=cpc&gclid=EAIaIQobChMI7Pm697G69QIV5tx
    MAh26AAKhEAAYASAAEgJSMfD_BwE

K.

https://www.stemcell.com/efficient-research/scientific-poster-presentations

https://www.scientifica.uk.com/neurowire/tips-for-presenting-your-scientific-poster-at-a-conference

[Unit 4]

Science Daily (2019) https://www.sciencedaily.com/releases/2019/04/190411101740.htm

Knowable Magazine (2019) https://knowablemagazine.org/article/mind/2019/psychological-effects-of-chronic-illness

Restricted Social Engagement among Adults Living with Chronic Conditions. Meek et al. (2018) https://www.ncbi.nlm.nih.gov/pmc/articles/PMC5800257/

Wikman et. al. PubMed (2011) https://pubmed.ncbi.nlm.nih.gov/21559485/

[Unit 5]

F.

https://www.roche.com/research_and_development/what_we_are_working_on/oncology/9_things_cancer.htm

https://www.mayoclinic.org/diseases-conditions/cancer/symptoms-causes/syc-20370588

https://www.cancer.org/cancer/cancer-basics/history-of-cancer/what-is-cancer.html

https://www.cancer.gov/about-cancer/causes-prevention/risk

https://www.cancer.net/navigating-cancer-care/prevention-and-healthy-living/understanding-cancer-risk

https://www.mayoclinic.org/diseases-conditions/cancer/symptoms-causes/syc-20370588

https://www.mayoclinic.org/tests-procedures/cancer-treatment/about/pac-20393344

https://www.mayoclinichealthsystem.org/locations/mankato/services-and-treatments/oncology/medical-oncology

https://www.nippon.com/en/japan-data/h01044/

https://genesenvironment.biomedcentral.com/articles/10.1186/s41021-016-0043-y

G.

https://www.narayanahealth.org/lung-cancer

K.

https://www.slideteam.net/blog/using-images-in-presentations-11-dos-and-donts

[Unit 6]

F.

https://www.mentalhealth.org.uk/a-to-z/s/stress

https://www.healthline.com/health/stress#types

https://www.stress.org/stress-effects

https://www.nimh.nih.gov/health/publications/stress

https://www.mayoclinic.org/healthy-lifestyle/stress-management/in-depth/stress-management/art-20044151

Engelmann, Julia " Number of suicides related to problems at work in Japan from 2010 to 2019," Statista, 6 April, 2020, https://www.statista.com/statistics/622325/japan-work-related-suicides/ accessed August 2021

https://www.statista.com/statistics/622325/japan-work-related-suicides/

[Unit 7]

F.

https://thesleepcharity.org.uk/information-support/adults/

https://www.sleepfoundation.org

https://www.mayoclinic.org/diseases-conditions/sleep-disorders/symptoms-causes/syc-20354018

https://my.clevelandclinic.org/health/articles/11429-common-sleep-disorders

https://www.nigms.nih.gov/education/fact-sheets/Pages/circadian-rhythms.aspx

https://en.wikipedia.org/wiki/Sleep

K.

https://bigfishpresentations.com/2012/07/20/preparing-presentations-5-ways-to-practice-til-perfect/

[Unit 8]

F.

https://americanaddictioncenters.org

https://newchoicestc.com

https://addictions.iu.edu

https://www.frontiersin.org/journals/psychiatry/sections/addictive-disorders

https://drugfree.org

https://drugabusestatistics.org/

https://academic.oup.com/bioscience/article/49/7/513/236613?login=false

https://www.mayoclinic.org/diseases-conditions/drug-addiction/symptoms-causes/syc-20365112

K.

https://www.nedarc.org/tutorials/utilizingdata/provideTakeHomeMessage.html

https://www.effectivepresentations.com/blog/handling-audience-questions/

https://business.tutsplus.com/tutorials/presentation-questions-answers-session--cms-35670

[Unit 9]

Alzheimer's Research UK. (2021). https://www.alzheimersresearchuk.org/about-us/how-we-do-it/big-initiatives/prevention

Strategies for dementia prevention: latest evidence and implications (2017)
https://www.ncbi.nlm.nih.gov/pmc/articles/PMC5546647/

Mediterranean Diet, Alzheimer Disease Biomarkers, and Brain Atrophy in Old Age (2021)
https://n.neurology.org/content/96/24/e2920

K.

https://www.nedarc.org/tutorials/utilizingdata/provideTakeHomeMessage.html

[Unit 10]

Extensions

https://www.drugs.com/slideshow/penicillin-wonder-drug-1215

https://knoema.com/atlas/Japan/topics/Demographics/Mortality/Infant-mortality-rate

https://embryo.asu.edu/pages/congenital-rubella-syndrome-crs

https://www.jpeds.or.jp/uploads/files/2020%20English%20JPS%20Immunization%20Schedule.pdf

F.

Totora, G.J, Grabowski, S.R. Principles of Anatomy & Physiology. 7th ed. New York: Harper Collins College Publishers; 1993.

https://www.history.com/topics/world-war-i/1918-flu-pandemic

https://www.mayoclinic.org/diseases-conditions/infectious-diseases/expert-answers/infectious-disease/faq-20058098

https://www.historyextra.com/period/medieval/history-hand-washing-how-when-start-past-disease/

https://www.acs.org/content/acs/en/pressroom/newsreleases/2008/june/pfizers-work-on-penicillin-for-world-war-ii-becomes-a-national-historic-chemical-landmark.html

https://www.jica.go.jp/english/our_work/thematic_issues/water/handwashing/index.html

https://www.jica.go.jp/english/news/field/2021/20211015_02.html
https://www.news-medical.net/health/History-of-Tuberculosis.aspx
https://www.ncbi.nlm.nih.gov/pmc/articles/PMC6518835/
https://www.who.int/news-room/fact-sheets/detail/influenza-(seasonal)
https://www.cdc.gov/plague/maps/index.html
https://www.reuters.com/world/asia-pacific/japan-reports-first-bird-flu-outbreak-season-culling-143000-chickens-2021-11-10/
https://www.healthline.com/health-news/seriously-dont-worry-about-the-plague#Heres-how-the-plague-spreads
https://www.med.or.jp/english/pdf/2003_09/390_400.pdf
https://www.who.int/news-room/fact-sheets/detail/tuberculosis
https://www.hotelmize.com/blog/quantifying-travel-how-many-people-travel-a-year/#How_Many_People_Traveled_Internationally_in_2019
https://www.cdc.gov/onehealth/basics/zoonotic-diseases.html

Research
https://www.britannica.com/science/bacteria
https://www.britannica.com/search?query=virus
https://www.khanacademy.org/science/biology/biology-of-viruses/virus-biology/a/intro-to-viruses
https://www.mayoclinic.org/diseases-conditions/tonsillitis/symptoms-causes/syc-20378479

I
https://www.ncbi.nlm.nih.gov/pmc/articles/PMC7874133/

J
https://www.webmd.com/cold-and-flu/what-is-flu
https://www.ncbi.nlm.nih.gov/pmc/articles/PMC7123171/

Discussion
https://www.britannica.com/event/1957-flu-pandemic
https://www.euro.who.int/en/health-topics/communicable-diseases/influenza/pandemic-influenza/past-pandemics
https://www.healthdirect.gov.au/what-is-a-pandemic
https://theconversation.com/coronavirus-b-cells-and-t-cells-explained-141888
https://www.frontiersin.org/articles/10.3389/fimmu.2019.01787/full
https://study.com/academy/lesson/what-is-the-lymphatic-system-structures-function-vocabulary.html

Diagram
https://socratic.org/questions/is-the-lymphatic-system-the-same-as-the-immune-system-are-both-of-these-terms-us

[Unit 11]
https://www.mayoclinic.org/diseases-conditions/amyotrophic-lateral-sclerosis/symptoms-causes/syc-20354022
https://pubmed.ncbi.nlm.nih.gov/29845377/
https://www.uclahealth.org/u-magazine/stem-cell-therapy-holds-promise-for-eliminating-hiv-infection
https://www.webmd.com/a-to-z-guides/symptoms-of-mononucleosis
https://www.mayoclinic.org/diseases-conditions/mononucleosis/symptoms-causes/syc-20350328
https://www.cdc.gov/hiv/basics/whatishiv.html
https://www.genome.gov/genetics-glossary/Retrovirus
https://www.who.int/health-topics/hiv-aids#tab=tab_1
https://www.nature.com/articles/s41598-020-75182-7
https://www.niid.go.jp/niid/en/865-iasr/10489-488te.html
https://japanhealthinfo.com/std-test/
https://www.nippon.com/en/japan-topics/c06603/misplaced-modesty-hampers-sex-education-in-japan's-schools.html
https://www.uclahealth.org/u-magazine/stem-cell-therapy-holds-promise-for-eliminating-hiv-infection
https://www.medicalnewstoday.com/articles/stem-cell-treatment-may-have-cured-woman-of-hiv
https://www.medicalnewstoday.com/articles/323893#transmission
https://www.medicalnewstoday.com/articles/is-there-a-cure-for-hiv#types
https://www.canberratimes.com.au/story/6750787/how-australia-tackled-the-aids-crisis/
https://www.upi.com/Science_News/2004/12/03/Japan-teens-have-high-STD-infection-rate/90051102069079/
https://www.webmd.com/sexual-conditions/ss/slideshow-std-pictures-and-facts
https://www.statista.com/statistics/870049/japan-hiv-infected-patients-by-gender/
https://www.asahi.com/ajw/articles/13978907
https://www.jmaj.jp/detail.php?id=10.31662%2Fjmaj.2021-0174
https://www.aidsmap.com/about-hiv/life-expectancy-people-living-hiv
https://www.mayoclinic.org/diseases-conditions/sexually-transmitted-diseases-stds/symptoms-causes/syc-20351240
https://medlineplus.gov/lab-tests/cd4-lymphocyte-count/
http://www.bccdc.ca/resource-gallery/Documents/Educational%20Materials/Epid/Other/CookersQA_Mar182010_.pdf
https://www.unaids.org/en/resources/presscentre/pressreleaseandstatementarchive/2022/february/20220211_Montagnier
https://www.unaids.org/en/resources/presscentre/pressreleaseandstatementarchive/2022/february/20220207_hiv-variant

https://www.hiv.gov/hiv-basics/staying-in-hiv-care/other-related-health-issues/opportunistic-infections

https://www.medicinenet.com/what_are_the_top_10_stds/article.htm

https://www.healthline.com/health/is-mono-an-std#contagious

https://www.mayoclinic.org/diseases-conditions/sexually-transmitted-diseases-stds/in-depth/std-symptoms/art-20047081

https://www.abc.net.au/news/2021-01-27/sex-education-lgbt-sexuality-young-high-school-pleasure-respect/12960062

https://nursing.usc.edu/blog/americas-sex-education/#legislation

https://www.aidsmap.com/news/feb-2022/one-person-remains-undetectable-without-hiv-drugs-almost-four-years-after-using

https://www.cdc.gov/hiv/basics/livingwithhiv/treatment.html

https://hivinfo.nih.gov/understanding-hiv/fact-sheets/hiv-medicines-and-side-effects

https://www.healthline.com/health/sexually-transmitted-diseases

https://www.acs.org/content/acs/en/education/whatischemistry/landmarks/flemingpenicillin.html

https://news.weill.cornell.edu/news/2022/02/patient-possibly-cured-of-hiv-infection-by-special-stem-cell-transplant

http://blog.futurefocusedlearning.net/10-steps-teaching-online-research-skills

[Unit 12]
F.

https://www.betterhealth.vic.gov.au/health/conditionsandtreatments/food-allergy-and-intolerance

https://medlineplus.gov/ency/article/000821.htm

https://www.carolinaasthma.com/blog/what-causes-a-person-to-develop-allergies/

https://www.mayoclinic.org/diseases-conditions/anaphylaxis/symptoms-causes/syc-20351468

https://www.mayoclinic.org/diseases-conditions/allergies/in-depth/allergy/art-20049365

https://www.goodto.com/wellbeing/top-natural-hay-fever-remedies-43399

https://blog.gaijinpot.com/strange-story-hay-fever-japan/

I.

https://blog.gaijinpot.com/strange-story-hay-fever-japan/

K.

https://ethos3.com/what-to-do-with-your-hands-during-presentations/

[Unit 13]

https://www.rsm.ac.uk/latest-news/2021/confronting-the-health-challenges-of-climate-change

https://www.who.int/heli/risks/ehindevcoun/en/

https://www.who.int/heli/risks/ehindevcoun/en/index2.html

https://www.ipcc.ch/sr15/

https://www.worldwildlife.org/threats/effects-of-climate-change

https://ec.europa.eu/clima/climate-change/causes-climate-change_en

K.

https://www.effectivepresentations.com/blog/handling-audience-questions/

https://business.tutsplus.com/tutorials/presentation-questions-answers-session--cms-35670

[Unit 14]
F.

Institute of Medicine (US) Committee on the Use of Complementary and Alternative Medicine by the American Public.
Washington (DC): National Academies Press (US); 2005.

Fjær, E.L., Landet, E.R., McNamara, C.L. et al. The use of complementary and alternative medicine (CAM) in Europe. BMC
Complement Med Ther 20, 108 (2020). https://doi.org/10.1186/s12906-020-02903-w

Origins and History of Chiropractic. https://www.acatoday.org/about/history-of-chiropractic/

Busse, J.W., Pallapothu, S., Vinh, B. et al. Attitudes towards chiropractic: a repeated cross-sectional survey of Canadian family physicians. BMC Fam
Pract22, 188 (2021). https://doi.org/10.1186/s12875-021-01535-4

Pan SY, Litscher G, Gao SH, et al. Historical perspective of traditional indigenous medical practices: the current renaissance and conservation of herbal
resources. Evid Based Complement Alternat Med. 2014;2014:525340. doi:10.1155/2014/525340

RMIT (Royal Melbourne Institute of Technology) https://www.rmit.edu.au/search?q=Chinese%20Medicine

https://www.australiangeographic.com.au/topics/history-culture/2011/02/top-10-aboriginal-bush-medicines/

https://www.engvid.com/vocabulary-advantages-disadvantages/

Language Advice

https://www.merriam-webster.com/thesaurus/

G.

https://www.nature.com/articles/nri148

I.

"National Institutes of Health (NIH) studies have shown that acupuncture is an effective treatment alone or in combination with conventional therapies."
https://www.hopkinsmedicine.org/health/wellness-and-prevention/acupuncture

K.

https://blog.prezi.com/zoom-presentation-tips/

https://www.youtube.com/watch?v=Uo0Wg3OD4Nc

CLILヘルス・エクスプラレイションズ

2023年 2 月20日　第 1 版発行

著　　　者——Chad L. Godfrey（チャド・L・ゴッドフリー）
　　　　　　Lauren Anderson（ローレン・アンダーソン）
　　　　　　Frances Gleeson（フランセス・グレーソン）
　　　　　　Stephen O'Toole（スティーブン・オトゥール）
　　　　　　Gautam Deshpande MD（ゴータマ・デシュパンデ）
　　　　　　種田佳紀（おいだ　よしき）
発　行　者——前田俊秀
発　行　所——株式会社 三修社
　　　　　　〒150-0001東京都渋谷区神宮前 2-2-22
　　　　　　TEL03-3405-4511　FAX03-3405-4522
　　　　　　振替 00190-9-72758
　　　　　　https://www.sanshusha.co.jp
　　　　　　編集担当　永尾真理
印刷・製本——日経印刷株式会社

©2023 Printed in Japan　ISBN978-4-384-33523-1 C1082

表紙デザイン——やぶはなあきお
本文DTP　　——川原田良一
イラスト　　——パント大吉
準拠音声録音——ELEC（英語教育協議会）
準拠音声製作——高速録音株式会社
準拠音声吹込——Jack Merluzzi / Rachel Walzer